"Yet another powerful contribution from McKenzie-Mavinga which offers a transformative framework for therapists, individuals and groups navigating the complex emotional landscape of antiblack racism. Using insight from decades of experience, she skilfully weaves personal narratives with professional wisdom, presenting a necessary and timely approach to healing. This book not only challenges traditional ideas of empathy but invites us all to embark on a journey of self-awareness, growth, and compassionate action. Essential reading for anyone dedicated to fostering authentic healing and dismantling racism."

Rotimi Akinsete, *Founder & Director, Black Men on the Couch*

"Dr Isha Mckenzie-Mavinga places the central theme of anti-Black racism—the distortion of perception and empathy by white individuals, front and centre in this comprehensive commentary of her life's work. She powerfully weaves her own experience, and the experience of many others involved in her work into a transformative call to action for anyone striving to create an anti-racist world."

Eugene Ellis, *Author of* Transforming Race Conversations:
A Healing Guide for Us All

"Dr Isha Mckenzie-Mavinga's life work illuminates the process of a black Empathic Approach as a model to heal the recursive life cycle of therapists navigating racialised hurts, slurs, and actions within the circumference and interior of the clients and institutions they work with. It is a must-have companion as a trilogy to the author's two former books. This masterpiece compassionately saves the black psyche from imploding into self-disruption and lovingly makes a stand for self-dignity, knowledge, and empowerment."

Karen Carberry, *Head of Family & Systemic Therapy, Orri, UK;*
Visiting Lecturer, University of Oxford, Doctorate in Clinical
Psychology Programme

I0025062

A Black Empathic Approach to Psychotherapy

This book presents the concept of a black Empathic Approach, an experiential model used as a means of developing powerful feelings associated with racism, such as fear, guilt, and rage, into a useful THERAPEUTIC tool for healing the intersectional impact of anti-black racism and associated oppressions.

Providing a framework for training, continued professional development, and therapeutic client work, this book explains the concept of the black Empathic Approach and discusses its usefulness in addressing racialization in a therapeutic context. It helps readers to unpick their use of empathy as a generic concept and develop it as a skill that can be used to assist others in addressing the trauma and impact of racism. Through a series of honest and transparent personal vignettes, Dr. McKenzie-Mavinga shares her own learning experience and personal growth from feelings of rage about racism to developing the approach and transforming pain into compassion. Chapters support processing, engagement and dialogue with contexts of anti-black racism in psychotherapy and counsellor training to provide a powerful framework for therapeutic discussion, teaching, learning and practice.

This book is intended for therapists, coaches, support workers, social workers, training institutes, and anyone else attempting to support individuals and groups impacted by racism.

Dr. Isha Mckenzie-Mavinga, Retired Psychotherapist, poet and lecturer, has thirty-three years' experience as a Transcultural Psychotherapist, Supervisor, Lecturer, Writer and Reiki Master. She contributed papers and poetry to several anthologies. Isha initiated therapeutic services at the African Caribbean Mental Health Association in Brixton, and at Women's Trust, working with women impacted by violence in relationships. She was a student counsellor and senior lecturer at London Metropolitan University and taught at Goldsmiths University of London. She has presented Black Issues workshops, based on concepts created during her Doctoral research and published in her books. As her legacy, she presents talks and trains master facilitators to present her concept of a black Empathic Approach to expand thinking and practice that embrace an emergence from the impact of racism and develop intersectional, anti-oppressive therapeutic practice in Counselling & Psychotherapy, psychology, and the caring professions.

A Black Empathic Approach to Psychotherapy

Growing from Rage to Compassion

Dr. Isha Mckenzie-Mavinga

Routledge
Taylor & Francis Group

LONDON AND NEW YORK

Designed cover image: The cover artwork is a painting created by
Dr. Isha Mckenzie-Mavinga, 2024, as an of expression of empathy towards the
misogynoir and silencing of Diane Abbot in parliament

First published 2026
by Routledge
4 Park Square, Milton Park, Abingdon, Oxon OX14 4RN

and by Routledge
605 Third Avenue, New York, NY 10158

Routledge is an imprint of the Taylor & Francis Group, an informa business

British Library Cataloguing-in-Publication Data
A catalogue record for this book is available from the British Library

ISBN: 9781032767666 (hbk)
ISBN: 9781032767628 (pbk)
ISBN: 9781003479994 (ebk)

DOI: 10.4324/9781003479994

Typeset in Times New Roman
by Newgen Publishing UK

Contents

Foreword

The trauma of anti-black racism goes back centuries. I wonder what it might have been like if my ancestors could have experienced Dr. Isha McKenzie-Mavinga's black Empathic Approach: being met with deep empathy, understanding and compassion for all that they experienced, and how the approach may have helped in perhaps some small (or big) way to ease or heal their traumatic experiences and rage. I reflect here about more recent times, where in my lifetime thus far, black individuals and communities have and continue to experience the trauma of anti-black racism, with threads of injustice weaved within and throughout. Anti-black racism is on the rise, and structural, systemic, and institutional racism continue to oppress black people in a myriad of ways. In the times that we are living now, the black Empathic Approach to psychotherapy is very much welcomed and needed.

In this remarkable book, an impressive interweave of personal and professional, Dr. Isha McKenzie-Mavinga offers us a way. No longer needing to hide behind the psychoanalytical/psychodynamic framework of the blank screen, this book illuminates brightly her courage, deep personal reflection and raw honesty as she journeyed from rage – towards a more compassionate self. The words of Maya Angelou come to mind here, 'And still I rise', and Dr. Isha McKenzie-Mavinga did indeed rise. Through her fierce determination and pioneering life's work as a leading transcultural psychotherapist, she offers us the black Empathic Approach: an approach she has developed over the last three decades that transcends therapeutic modality and can be used by *all* therapists of *all* modalities

Whilst tracing her own transformation of powerful feelings, namely rage, she shares aspects of her journey and the context of developing empathy. Equally, by critiquing and building on the concept, one of the 'necessary and sufficient' conditions for therapeutic change to occur, Dr. Isha Mckenzie-Mavinga challenges us to consider whether we can subjectively *'see, think and feel'* as the other in relation to anti-black racism. For healing to occur, she rightly argues that we can no longer accept the taken for granted stance about empathy and the assumption that as humans, we are all naturally empathic. As recent research and lived experience accounts of therapy have revealed, much harm has been done to black clients in the therapy room when sharing their experiences of racism (Samuel, 2023). Much harm also continues to be caused to black students in counselling and psycho-therapy training as well.

Breathing new life into the concept of empathy, Dr. Isha McKenzie-Mavinga also asks us to not only (re)consider our own empathic abilities and responses in relation to anti-black racism, but also to whiteness. In the first chapter 'Breaking through colour blindness', we are gifted with a powerful account of the black Empathic Approach *in action*, reflecting the specialness and uniqueness in its ability to extend to white individuals who are willing to explore their whiteness. A deeper dive into white privilege and the defensiveness that perpetuates anti-black racism is further explored in the noteworthy chapter 'Being white hurts'. What these two chapters teach us, is that a willingness to engage in anti-racist work is essential and the need to transform our empathic understandings of the trauma of anti-black racism, crucial. For those of us who are willing, Dr. Isha Mckenzie-Mavinga invites us – on both sides – to lean into the black Empathic Approach as a means of elevating our emotional and psychological well-being.

Each and every chapter in this book is an open invitation to unravel and create new ravellings: the nuances of 'an appropriate gaze', the context surrounding internalised racism, and the intersections of oppressions that black women experience, to name but a few. In the particularly poignant chapter 'Unburied and undried tears', we gain a transgenerational understanding that connects the potency of history not laid to rest, hovering in the ancestral domain and psyche. Through the reading of this book, one incredible chapter after the other, ultimately, we will learn that identifying and addressing our rage as a feature of personal development towards compassion, is the key element in the use of the black Empathic Approach.

Dr. Isha McKenzie-Mavinga's trailblazing thirty-year career and significant contribution to the field of counselling and psychotherapy has been nothing short of revolutionary. This, alongside her two inspirational books, *Black Issues in the Therapeutic Process* (2009) and *The Challenge of Racism in Therapeutic Practice* (2016) have paved the way for many of us to follow. Standing on her shoulders and alongside in sisterhood, I am honoured to write this foreword for this, her third 'legacy' book, and to call Isha my friend.

Helen P. George

Psychotherapist, Founder of Community Trauma UK and host of its bi-annual conference, PhD Researcher, and editor of *Black Women, Trauma and Therapy: Revolutionising Therapeutic Thought and Practice* (2025)

Acknowledgements

My deepest respect and gratitude to all who have journeyed alongside me throughout the gestation and birthing of this project: BAATN, Eugene Ellis, Jayakara Ellis. Helen George, Sharon Jennings, Thelma Perkins, Laureen Burris-Phillips, Caroline Alexis, Joanne John. Karen Carberry, Rotimi Akinsete, Aileen Alleyne, Anne Remy, Leah Thorn, Wendy Francis, Hyacinth Fraser, Nicole Turner, Dee Morrison, Lydia Purichelli, Phoenix Gentiles, Liz Mitchell, Sharon Hastings, Denise Lyttle & My Children & Grans.

Also, gratitude and thanks to those who supported the concept, trusted in my work and facilitated workshops: Gloria Boadi, Umaa Thampu, , Moriam Grillo, Lexi Noel, Amanda Crutchley, Pauline Miller, Nerissa Mcdonald, Robert Sookhan, Kemi Omijeh, Mary Pascall, Shally Gadhoke, , Pauline Miller,, Nikita Constant, .

Introduction

A black Empathic Approach requires the therapeutic skill of emotional connection, a shared context of the impact of racism and empathic responses built around awareness of self, in relation to intersecting oppressions, socio-cultural silencing and the institutional and personal impact of anti-black racism. These words are expressed from reality and the experience of applying the concept during Psychotherapy and training.

During my research, I became aware of how rage features as one of the powerful feelings attached to reflecting on the effect of anti-black racism. I coined the term 'Recognition trauma' to offer a framework for therapists when working with powerful feelings attached to racism. From this recognition, emerged other useful concepts, and the knowledge that compassion, creativity, courage and congruence, are necessary ingredients when interacting with individuals and groups regarding the impact of racism. I do not feel that I am able to prescribe a solution to the mental and physical impact of anti-black racism, however, I am aware that many authors are carrying forward this work about understanding themselves and the relationships that either perpetuate or assist in healing the impact of racism.

Writing about this concept helps me to realise that examining the development of my own rage and compassion opens a door for promoting the use of a black Empathetic Approach to Psychotherapy. A dynamic recognition of the emotions of black people and people of colour (BPOC) is key to this process.

I present this approach as a framework for the relational process when working with racism in therapeutic contexts. This model can also be thought about in terms of working therapeutically with other oppressions. Although useful as a component of working with anti-black racism, it is important to accept that empathy with the oppression of anti-black racism is not the same as empathy with other oppressions. One cannot claim to know the experience and personal context of anti-black racism because you have an experience of sexism, homophobia, or ableism.

Hurts associated with direct oppression and covert oppression may be similar, but they are not the same. Anti-black racism was designed to divide and subjugate people with black and brown skins, of different shades and hair textures, other than straight and blond.

DOI: 10.4324/9781003479994-1

Of course, this experience intersects with other oppressions. We cannot therefore simply transfer our offerings of empathy about one hurtful oppression to another. This has shown up as a confused response emerging in some of the workshops based on my former books. 'Black issues in the Therapeutic Process' (2009) and 'The Challenge of Racism in Therapeutic Practice' (2016).

This book presents an autobiographical approach to exploring the challenges that professionals experience when considering therapeutic engagement with the process of anti-black racism. As an example of developing a black Empathic Approach to psychotherapy, I present personal vignettes of my life process and personal development influences, while transforming my rage into a more compassionate self.

During workshops presenting a black Empathic Approach to Psychotherapy, individuals have felt challenged to extend their understanding of empathy as traditionally taught. Naïve participants expected their empathic offerings would be sufficient for this task and were surprised at the challenge to look deeper at their relationship with anti-black racism and the defences that this can trigger.

Whilst presenting my personal life experiences of rage, and my process of harnessing compassion, the book offers a complimentary approach to the use of empathy in the context of anti-black racism and its impact on individuals.

This is a book for therapists, support workers, Psychologists, social workers, training institutes, those in humanist professions and lay persons wanting to build an anti-racist world. It is a journey through training experiences of those who have dared to accept that anti-black racism is damaging to the psyche of all peoples, and those who have dared to imagine that the veiled silence of individuals and institutions can be lifted.

The book presents a culmination of thirty years of work in the field of psychotherapy and counselling. It portrays insights from workshops, talks, and dynamic interactions that address the impact of anti-black racism. It offers consideration of diversity and sameness and the ethical consequences of ignoring the impact of anti-black racism on identity and personal development. It invites readers to engage with the idea that we all have the potential to process, evaluate and emerge from oppressions that may have shut us down and created low self-esteem and voicelessness.

The book promises an ethical commitment to black lives matter and the emergence of black minds from the trauma of racism. It is an invitation to merge the political with personal and psychological, in therapeutic relationships. Most importantly, I share my journey as a psychotherapist, researcher, writer and person of colour.

I feel compelled to share with readers my original choice of a title. 'A black Empathic Approach / Growing Through Rage about Racism to Compassion and an Appropriate Gaze'. It turns out that the proposition of 'an appropriate gaze' became absorbed into the book and held its own in Chapter 7. An appropriate gaze means harnessing ways of therapeutic modelling that challenge anti-black racism and support the hurt rather than silencing or perpetuating it.

It is my hope that readers will become aware that to present a black Empathic Approach to Psychotherapy, it is necessary to address rage about racism and adopt a compassionate attitude. This is the glue that reinforces an appropriate gaze, robust enough to work with this concept.

Throughout the book, the initials BPOC, will be used to identify black and people of colour. The initials BEAP will be used for a black Empathic Approach to Therapy. I use lowercase 'b' for the term 'black'. This supports the meaning of this term in a political sense (denoting those impacted by anti-black racism, and not intended to describe a skin colour).

Transparency

Readers will notice that I have been transparent, in describing some personal experiences that show the process of my journey prior to and throughout writing this book. I decided it was important to share some areas of my life that reach beyond being a psychotherapist and have supported a life process throughout the development of a black Empathic Approach to Psychotherapy. This approach dispels the mythology of human perfection, behind the screen of a psychotherapist. We are taught to be a blank screen while in practice. I am now retired from practice and having held this protocol and the power that goes with it, for thirty plus years, I feel it is time to show myself.

About me

I want to tell you about where this perspective of a 'black Empathic Approach to psychotherapy came from, and how it's been growing over the past twenty-five years since my initial research and practice with professionals, trainees, students, supervisees and clients.

I first realised that I was a counsellor when I was a youth worker in a community centre, not far from my home, in Southeast London. I noticed that the young black boys would sit down and talk to me when they came to the coffee bar to buy snacks and drinks. They would talk to me about their family lives, and what was going on in the neighbourhood and how they were feeling. That was my first realisation that I had good listening skills, apart from being a mother.

Then after that, I went to work in a community project where long-term unemployed people were being retrained to go back into the employment market. There was a lot of diversity, including people with disabilities and minority sexualities. People who had experienced a rough time not being at work for many years. My job title was 'Outreach Worker'. I was supposed to assist individuals to come into the project and talk about how they feel and make decisions about what they wanted to learn to get them back on the road to employment. Once again, I was listening and supporting in the best way I knew how.

Then a new colleague, a black woman, came into the project. She had worked in mental health for a few years previously, and she was given the job of Counsellor.

People started talking to her, who had previously been speaking to me. So now there were two black women, and I thought she had come in and taken my job. Then I thought, well I need to make something of this and that was when I spoke to a friend, who recommended the institute where I could train as a counsellor. I decided, I'm going to train and then I'll get a job like hers, with a title.

I wasn't given a place on the training course immediately. They wanted me to go on a part-time course and although I wasn't happy, I went on it. I said ok it's knock, knock, I want you to let me in the front door this time. I went back and eventually they let me in. It was a three-year postgraduate diploma in Psychodynamic Counselling which was equivalent to a psychotherapy training.

I was challenged by my training, as the only person of colour and I felt marginalised in a predominantly white institution that refused to give attention to my experience as a black woman, and what was needed to acknowledge and use racial identity as something that could be worked with in a therapeutic exchange.

I was not very happy there, but I went through with it. We had the opportunity to see clients on the premises and to have our supervision on the premises. I felt that everything was controlled, colonised and institutionalised.

The training institution was situated in a largely white affluent area of London serving mostly white clients. I noticed they had this book where they registered clients' details. Alongside some client's names were written, 'West Indian' or 'African' and I'd think, oh maybe I can work with this person. They put their names in the back of the book because they assumed that these client's situations were complex and needed senior therapists. They used the word 'borderline mental health' and that really got my back up. I was never offered any black clients, and I used to speak my truth during class and supervision meetings, which were led by white lecturers and supervisors.

Everything was internal. I was a black woman working with white clients. Being sensitive to racial diversity, I wanted to explore the nuances of offering therapy to clients similar and very different to me. I also felt I'd have more to offer black clients, based on some of the racism they may have experienced, which was intersectional to their lives. That was in 1985. I was seen as a bit weird, because I was challenging the system that wasn't facilitating my own learning as a black woman. After that I practised as a Psychotherapist for about thirty-three years, and that includes twenty-six years of higher education teaching on Counselling and Psychotherapy courses, private practice and as a student counsellor.

After my training, I worked at the African Caribbean Mental Health Association in Brixton. The staff were all black African, Caribbean and people of colour. The team consisted of a director, a solicitor, a housing worker, a volunteer befriending worker, administrator and liaison person. The staff team worked, inside and outside of the local mental Health hospitals, with people who were at risk of going into a Psychiatric hospital and those who had been sectioned under the Mental Health Act.

There was a lot to understand and deal with in terms of offering them a familiar face, because many of them had experienced Police prejudice and racial harassment that had been ignored. One woman was locked up for singing loudly on her balcony.

Previously, there had been no real counselling and therapeutic space in the project to consider and share their experiences. Effectively the clients were victims of a revolving door system, which meant detainment, sectioning under the Mental Health Act, homelessness and hospitalisation. The challenge was to put something in place as an alternative, to prevent hospitalisation, or to support after hospitalisation. Many clients were enraged about how unfairly they were being treated within the system. I had enough fire in my belly to initiate a supportive team of therapists, who could offer an appropriate gaze and a black Empathic Approach to Psychotherapy. This is where it all began.

My research kicked off when I became a senior lecturer at a university in London. I also attended two other universities to support tutors to think about changing their attitudes and to assist students to think differently about learning and practice that acknowledges and addresses the impact of anti-black racism.

This book has been written in two places where I live and belong. The first is England where I grew up and the second Trinidad & Tobago, my father's ancestral home.

Tobago 2020

The rainy season has been long and arduous. We have been experiencing flash flooding, landslides and economic and environmental concerns. For the last six weeks I have been mainly confined to the home, resting and recovering from arriving and making a greater effort to listen to my body and create spiritual, emotional, and physical balance daily. My life has slowed, chores take longer, and night comes faster. This feels like a rite of passage.

We are two decades into the Millennium and diseases such as Lupus, Thalassemia, and Sickle cell are rarely given the time of day. A belated announcement has been made, that medication for sickle cell sufferers is now on the market. I can't help thinking that the diseases effecting people with melanin, have been marginalised and may be a silent genocide, perpetuated by racism.

Elderhood, womanhood and intersecting oppressions

There have also been downsides to my experience here in Tobago. I cannot deny that as a single older woman, my presence has attracted young local men searching for a cougar. This position of trying to break through poverty by latching on to a Westerner is common. I could be sitting quietly on a beach and a young man would come up to me and ask to be my friend. Sometimes they are married or already partnered, and this is a normal practice here. Recently a young man commented, 'you would have been just right for me when you were twenty-five' I don't believe he realised the impact of this remark on me as a senior and female. I am tired of pointing out racism, sexism, misogyny and downright disrespect from the men here. I kid myself I am retired from the battle, because I am doing less work directly related to racism, but I cannot deny the oppressions in my everyday life, so I have learned to respond with humour. Who wouldn't want to get close to a powerful, kind, loving, successful, black woman.

In 2012, during one of my workshops, A black man asked, 'do I think that racism can be eliminated?' my answer was 'no'. 'As with the trauma of all oppressions we must find ways to live with it and chip away at it, for our own self-preservation'. Although I have facilitated many workshops that address the trauma of racism, and practise ways to elevate ourselves from its impact, or from internalising the experience, I am aware that there is a lot of work to be done. Including work on shadism/colourism and internalised racism, within the BPOC community.

Whilst the white community addresses their privilege, black people and people of colour, need safe spaces to address our deliverance from the transgenerational, intersectional divisive impact of colonialism and slavery.

There is a high cost to being a woman of colour in the role of facilitator doing anti-racist work. We cannot underestimate re traumatisation and the vicarious trauma of holding groups whilst they wake from the silence of being unable to address the impact of anti-black racism, internalised racism and perpetrator positioning.

In 2023 the police force in Scotland, publicly admitted to being institutionally racist, sexist and misogynist. Though long overdue, this was a rare and welcome shift. Personal and institutional growth takes a lifetime and is a continuous process for individuals and the systems that perpetrate anti-black racism.

The workshops I have been running are a form of resistance to the damage that has been done and still needs to be addressed in terms of mental and physical well-being. I do not want resistance to kill me because that would be murder, or suicide, yet although I can retire from the battlefield, I cannot retire from resistance. I want to create a legacy for my work and sometimes the road is lonely. For this reason, I decided to use my voice and portray evidence and explanation of my journey to a much-needed concept. 'The black Empathic Approach' to Psychotherapy.

An anti-racist journey

An anti-racist journey is the practice of opposing racism and actively living the principles of challenging and working through the damage that racism can cause to body mind and spirit. I became concerned about this during my psychotherapy training, when I realised I was being affected by the trauma that racism causes, and the neglect of its impact on black minds. It was later that I became aware of how racism also damages white minds, bodies and souls.

This book embraces thought and action that moves towards healing the negative, intersectional, silent, enduring impact of anti-black racism. I have interweaved my personal story and reminiscence with academic thought and persuasion, in a way that is transparent to readers, thus showing the humanness of a black therapist's personal and professional journey and how I have lived the principle of a 'black

Empathic Approach' to Psychotherapy and healing the trauma that anti-black racism can cause. The concept will be abbreviated at times. (BEAP)

Chapter outlines

Chapter 1: Breaking through colour blindness

This chapter opens the book with the testimony of Anne, a white female supervisee and her learning experience. Fear and guilt about racism were met with compassion and a black Empathic Approach, during facilitation of my transcultural supervision group. The chapter also shares workshop experiences of learning and facilitation of a black Empathic Approach to Psychotherapy.

Chapter 2: The context and quality of empathy

This chapter reflects on the context and content of Empathy in generic, personal and psychological thinking. It describes my journey to understanding the use of empathy and my building of self to create robust attunement, that combines empathy with leaning into experiences of anti-black racism on individuals. I reflect on my personal experience of empathy from early days to adulthood.

Chapter 3: Breathing new life into empathy

This chapter encourages trust in personal ability to transform a one-dimensional approach to empathy, into something more specifically related to the context and concept of a black Empathic Approach, and healing anti-black racism. This means not taking empathy for granted, not relying on assumptions that as humans we are naturally empathic, and that the use of empathy is essentially generic. A willingness to transform responses to racism for the benefit of anti-racist work is required. The concept of a black Empathic Approach to Psychotherapy offers a framework for working with black issues in the therapeutic process, that cannot be matched with a taken for granted stance about empathy.

Chapter 4: Assimilation and humiliation

This chapter addresses the influences of heritage and assimilation, alongside cultural norms and humiliation. For some, rituals and cultural customs mark their entrance to the world. Language and the rules of citizenship, become a blueprint. As benign humans, we become impressed by limiting societal oppressions and the challenge of achieving prosperity and self-esteem. We learn that Assimilation can be closely linked to a sense of belonging, engendered or dispelled at an early age. Humiliation occurs with negative projections, stigmas and the oppressions, that unchecked, can keep us small. I share some of my journey and heritage experiences. The humiliation of Windrush migrants, rejection and repatriation is highlighted as an example of how institutional power can humiliate individuals, migrant communities, black people and people of colour.

Chapter 5: Engaging with internalised racism

This chapter addresses the cause of individuals struggling with the impact of anti-black racism. They often face denial and defensiveness from those around them and these responses exacerbate abnormal feelings in addition to the hurt of anti-black racism. If onlookers or perpetrators of racism are naive or rigidly protecting themselves from the challenge of this experience, they can act in ways that give the receiver cause to believe that there is something wrong with them. Lack of being believed, misinterpretation, or nowhere to process the wound causes internalised racism. I reflect on examples that present this dilemma, and how the use of a black Empathic Approach to Psychotherapy can support individuals to move through this.

Chapter 6: Being white hurts

This chapter offers insights and wisdom about turning defensiveness into compassion, a fundamental element for working with a black Empathic Approach to Psychotherapy. Being white hurts differently for a person of colour experiencing an attack aimed at them because they are other than white. There are similarities and differences in the pain experienced by a white person, a brown skinned person and a person whose heritage is associated with being black African or Asian. White fragility, a phenomenon now discussed more openly, has become a phase of personal development that white individuals encounter, when their privilege is confronted. This is why it is necessary to unpick colonial heritage underlying white responses to this challenge. Obviously, this cannot happen unless willingness to go there and sit with the pain and privilege of having a white skin occurs. In this chapter I present interview responses from a white colleague.

Chapter 7: Developing an appropriate gaze

In this chapter I make the case that an appropriate gaze is essential for the use of a black Empathic Approach. An appropriate gaze is a reflective process that accurately responds to and reflects the situation at hand. In the case of the BPOC group, or anyone, describing an experience of anti-black racism. This means reflection and appropriate modelling in the relational process. An appropriate gaze is one that positively reflects a connection with an individual's true identity and ways of being. Attention to internalised racism and its impact on BPOC individuals and the ways that anti-black racism distorts the perception of white individuals, is an essential part of the therapist's contribution to building an appropriate gaze.

Chapter 8: Unburied and undried tears

This chapter connects the potency of history not laid to rest, hovering in the ancestral domain and the psyche. The title draws on Nourbese Philip's (2017) presentation of the decimation of Identity, expressed through performance. (Talk-John Hope Franklin Humanities Institute, Duke University 8.8.2017.) With a deep guttural empathic resonance, she invokes the memory and sorrow of enslaved Africans on the Dutch ship 'Zong' in 1781, of whom 150 were thrown overboard and drowned, on the way to Jamaica so the ship's owners could collect the insurance. (Gregson v. Gilbert maritime insurance case 1783). '*Undried tears*' means sorrow, imprinted throughout generations, due to the trauma of anti-black racism. Phillips performs 'Zong' with a sacred reverence to the ancestors. She respectfully ritualises the '*Unburied*' and sense of ancestral grief 'undried tears'. There is a hush in the audience, as if rendered speechless, transported, into a frozen past. The silence of bodies Unburied, floating haplessly on the ocean of '*Undried Tears*'. In using the term 'undried tears', I am referring to lost opportunities to express the pain of anti-black racism, that this chapter will address. A black Empathic Approach is encouraged to process the feeling of being silenced that can fragment identity.

Chapter 9: Reclaiming the minds, we never lost

This chapter presents the idea that putting attention on reclaiming wellness and developing anti-racist approaches to mental well-being, is preferable to labelling expressions of frustration and rage about racism as madness. Persistent gaslighting as a response to a call for help about the impact of anti-black racism has been known to cause low self-esteem and concerns about mental ill health. My rationale for putting attention on this state comes from observing the impact of anti-black racism as an intersecting oppression on the whole self, including the mind. This suggests a form of trauma. The chapter highlights ways that reviewing empathic responses can enhance the capacity to respond to the trauma of racism and strengthen the mind.

Chapter 10: Black woman and self-care

This chapter highlights an important context for black women and the types of racism they face. A particular kind of black Empathic Approach that is intersectional and honouring to her experiences and internalised racism, sexism, and misogynoir is important. I emphasise the importance of not assuming that feminist theory fits all women and accepting that this context is vital to a black Empathic Approach to therapy. The chapter highlights the importance of remembering that our diverse experiences, due to skin colour and misogynoir are key elements in the psychology of black women, whether we deem ourselves to be feminist or not. I emphasise that the act of loving every part of ourselves is the essence of self-care.

Chapter 11: A work in progress

This chapter is a summary of my personal development throughout my journey of developing the concept of a black Empathic Approach to Psychotherapeutic practice. I present my experience of bringing forth ideas that come from within and support life and professional experience. I am neither here nor there, yet I have a sense of arrival. A completion, yet somehow a beginning, and I am still here, I still have a voice, and my mind is still intact. I have made the space and time to voice what I know as a unique contribution to the field of psychotherapy, counselling and relational thought. I value the freedom to show myself. To be transparent about my journey. I am a work in progress. This chapter expresses gratitude and shares the pros and cons of moving towards my legacy work. I am grateful for having had the opportunity to train a group of masters to carry forward the facilitation of a black Empathic Approach. I show the importance of sharing this work and passing it on.

Chapter 12: The legacy, a black Empathic Approach

This chapter summarises the legacy of my work promoting and modelling the concept of a black Empathic Approach. It is a framework for a psychotherapeutic dialogue about anti-black racism, whilst at the same time, an encouragement to share areas of personal development, essential to the cause of healing the mental and emotional damage that anti-black racism can create. This book shows that psychotherapists are real people with life stories. One that breaks away from the hierarchy of the therapist's role and demonstrates our humanness and personal challenges along the way. The chapters represent an engagement with the timeline of my life. A life of being British and building an acquaintance with my Caribbean heritage. I have shared some of my experiences and my deepest thoughts and personal development that have weaved into the creation of this legacy.

I conclude with an excerpt from Anne's interview with me and acknowledge this as an appropriate Gaze from a white therapist.

Chapter 1

Breaking through colour blindness

Colour blindness can start with disbelief that oppression exists. Many people live their lives as colour-blind and ignorant of the existence of other oppressions. A choice not to see or not to believe and, therefore, not to witness the experience at the receiving end of racism is personal, political and institutional. Whether this be lack of awareness, denial or unconscious ways of self-protection from engaging with the experience, this does not make the experience unreal. We must ask ourselves whether a decision not to engage with these experiences is useful.

Excerpt from Annewriting

'My name is Anne, and I am a racist, but I'm working on it, knowing that this is a lifelong process which has no finish line. If I truly want to commit to working on it, I have to explore the most uncomfortable parts of myself. I must be willing to lose privilege, comfort, stability, and my understanding of the way the world works. I'm not just a racist, by the way, I'm a homophobe, a transphobe, an ableist and ageist and a sexist. How could I not be? I'm a straight, cis, white woman with a powerful passport, who grew up in a world designed for people like me. For all intent and purpose, it's in my best interest to stop writing this essay now because succeeding in this world means that people like me have to lose out so that other people can win, or so I thought. My passion for anti-bigotry was largely a flagellating exercise fuelled by guilt and shame with the intention of making things better for others while martyring myself on the altar of privilege. Looking down from the ivory tower atop my moral high ground, I could shout the truth of wokeness to all the bigots below. I alone would atone for my millennia of justice by laying my comfort down for the comfort of others, sacrificing myself for the greater good. I could have easily spent my entire life like this. I sought ways to do more work and to affirm my suffering, which led me to Doctor Isha Mckenzie-Mavinga, who, instead of validating my guilt, offered me compassion.

Bigotry is fear. Holding onto fear only separates us from ourselves and from others; it is an unhealthy clinging that blocks self-exploration. In this way bigotry is a sickness of the majority we are desperately trying to cure by looking at the

DOI: 10.4324/9781003479994-2

symptoms, not the cause. Racism is the result of a "misplaced white gaze". Dr. Isha said to me. With that, I realised that I needed to turn inwards. Dr. Isha's invitation to explore my relationship with my whiteness led me to explore my need to be good and my inherent belief that I am bad. Her compassion reminded me that my sickness is worth healing, not just to save others, but to save myself. In my desire to be a healer, I forgot that I'm also worth being healed. In that respect, maybe I was right; People like me have to lose our fear so that everyone can win. From the beginning, I knew I would do my reflective inquiry on something involving my work with minority clients, but it was this exploration of my inherent belief that I am bad, that led me to my struggle to be seen as good. It was Dr. Isha's compassion that allowed me to ask myself how my need to be good was disproportionately affecting my minority clients?'

Anne was a supervisee who attended one of my transcultural supervision groups. Finding herself face to face with black peers in a supervision group, led by me, was a challenge. Not just a challenge for her co-supervisors but also a challenge for me as a black woman. A challenge to my use of the concept 'a black Empathic Approach' and its application to white individuals and groups.

I decided to present an excerpt from her reflective inquiry that she offered to the group when our meetings were ending, and I was preparing for retirement. The black women in the group had a thirst for recognition and transparency about the traumatic impact of racism on their work and their lives as counsellors and I was modelling a black Empathic Approach to Psychotherapy.

Not only was it a moving experience when Anne read her excerpt to the group, but it also spoke to me about my work, my authorship and my accomplishment of an aim to establish a black Empathic Approach as a conscious skill set in developing antiracist approaches to therapeutic work with anyone, be they BPOC or white, trainees, professional, therapist, supervisor or supervisee.

The challenge of devising a concept that creates an active approach to developing anti racist practice was not easy. Throughout the years of presenting workshops based on research and experience presented in my previous books, there were many peaks and troughs. I express deep gratitude to the individuals who wanted to further their understanding and application of this approach under my guidance.

This was also a realisation and practice setting for using the concept with white trainees and professionals willing to explore their whiteness and 'recognition trauma' and the powerful feelings, fears and defences that arose when racism was being considered and discussed in their learning settings, supervision and client work. This required them to give up their colour blindness and see their own whiteness in the context of how their skin colour privilege contributed to denial and perpetuated racism. An important element in doing this work was that of holding discussions without not leaning on black participants for their learning and whilst regarding the black participants' learning needs. This 'blaxplaining', and risk of tokenising has been a phenomenon in mixed racial groups and has resulted in further frustration and hurt to BPOC participants, whose powerful feelings are often not considered.

After a series of workshops, I asked some of the individuals who had experienced the workshops as participants and then been trained as facilitators by me, if they could reflect on their experience, of workshop participants internalising and overstanding the ways that this concept was being taken on board, or not as the case may be. They speak openly about their life experiences of the black Empathic Approach.

Here are some of the individual reflections about the approach.

GB: comments

My first experience of the black Empathic Approach was in the reading of, 'Black Issues in the Therapeutic Process (2009)'. My masters training with Dr. Isha brought more clarity. It seemed straightforward enough. I did not have much heightened emotions around the subject. However, it was in the role of a facilitator in a Challenge workshop, especially with predominantly white participants, that I found the power of the approach and the need for courage and persistence to be able to use the approach. It was not as straightforward as it had appeared, and participants tended to deflect and not focus on the actual concept. It appears that anything to do with race, especially 'blackness' causes people to become uncomfortable and not want to address it directly. There is a tendency to want to dilute it. There was also a tendency to focus on modalities and the personal style of the therapist. In the video clip, the example used in the training demonstrates the approach (Bernice/ Counselling about Shadism. (Alleyne, Tuckwell 2008). I found that there was the need to constantly refocus participants back to looking at the black Empathic Approach. Some of the defences from white participants at the start made me frustrated and angry but with experience and support from Dr. Isha, I have been able to address people's disrespect and bias with courage, humility, and compassion, explaining to participants in summary that the approach has to be viewed in terms of a framework for dialogue and clarity. They have to name racism in the room if it appears and they should not be afraid to explore differences. The black Empathic Approach encourages participants to address racism. Therapists might want to use a different approach, but if they are acknowledging black, multicultural issues and oppressions then they are in essence using a black Empathic Approach, so what they call it does not matter. I feel that the framework offers a safe but challenging approach that enables effective and compassionate therapy.

In my personal life as a therapist, I have integrated the Black Empathic Approach into my work with clients and it has been received with appreciation. I am sure that I have retained clients, and I have shown a greater understanding of their whole being including specific issues pertaining to racism. Not just because I am a black woman, but I am able to name the issue of racism, external and internal and blackness in the space as it appears.

My observations were not directly related to the challenge workshop, but rather based on comments from peers, tutors, and observations of skill sessions at university. For example: Student peers used avoidance statements such as "I don't see colour" and "I wait for the client to mention the differences between us and issues around racism".

UT: comments

A tutor in feedback of a skills session omitted cultural aspects as to why someone's non-verbal communications could be culturally related, i.e. No eye contact from certain groups. After a gentle challenge, the tutor was honest enough to say my challenge has helped him to bring more understanding of difference to his practice. While observing a skills session the student client was clearly distressed by the racism experienced at work. The therapist totally ignored the part that the client tried to bring into the space. The peer student counsellor reflected that she ignored the racism because she did not know what to do–lack of BEA!!!

There was a painful realisation in the Master Graduate facilitator workshop where my defences were brought to light in relation to a racist incident at an anti-racist workshop. A white colleague continued to interrupt the workshop by stating racist comments at a compulsory anti racism training e.g., 'George Floyd was a criminal', 'All Lives Matter etc'. My defences were going to my head, and I was intellectualising as a protective veering away from the feelings that arise from the impact of racism such as shame, a sense of isolation, and feeling abandoned. The film 'Get Out' (Peele 2017) has a powerful image of 'a Sunken Place'. The director, Peele explores 'sunken place' as a place where you feel that no matter how hard you scream you can't get your agency across. Racism interrupts and hijacks my sense of agency. I did not give consent to this attack on my body and psyche. The racist interruption steals my sense of focus and interrupts my learning. It robs me of my words and the ground beneath me gives way like falling into the 'sunken Place'. Racism is incredibly crazy making and discombobulating.

Dr. Isha slowed this down and challenged me appropriately by asking could my history of being a South Asian Tamil, brown bodied female be getting in the way of asking a black, African, female facilitator for help. Yes! (Mckenzie-Mavinga (2009. P70), 'individuals remain slightly invisible to themselves, defending against the fear of adverse attention. Therefore, the black client's developmental process can become overwhelmed by defence construction'.

My defences highlighted the internalised racism I was experiencing. I felt seen, held and challenged via the black Empathic Approach. It was illuminating to understand the layers of how racism interrupts my learning, my connection to my vulnerability and the difficulty and resistance that I had been articulating to a black colleague, can you help me please?

PM: comments

The black Empathic Approach acknowledges cultural differences in the therapeutic space. It enables openness for discussions around differences between Black/white dyads. The openness allows for exploration of expectations in the relationship based on differences. This includes checking why the Black client decided to see a white therapist and a black therapist for that matter. Diversity can be acknowledged with sensitive disclosure about differences. The BEA takes account of the assessment of experiences of racism and other forms of oppression. The therapist is encouraged to broach the subject of oppression and how the sessions could be used to address this.

The BEAP can also be mirrored in supervision to explore what it feels like to work with black issues. The BEAP enables the 'repositioning' of the white counsellor in a more proactive place of 'engaging their authentic self as well as the black client's whole self.' In essence, this could lead to improved psychological contact and experience, where there is a disconnect due to the unaddressed differences in therapeutic relationships. My own awareness of differences occurs every day, and I am challenged to process my internalised and intersecting hurts.

UK-July 2018

I am a single woman again. My partner of 11 years passed away. Since then, I've been very flat. It meant a lot to have a loyal black man beside me as a friend. Last night just as I placed my head on the pillow, I heard three knocks. It did not take long for him to visit me. One of my friends said that he came in on the Virgin Airlines that landed last night and took my friends back to England. He was one of three significant black men in my life. The first was my father, yet I cannot talk of a relationship as he passed away when I was four months old and was never replaced by a stepfather, or surrogate father. My relationships with black men remained an intangible mystery, until I became a mature woman, raising sons, when I decided it was time to learn more about men.

Discovering men and what it is to be a man, came with my first 'in love' relationship in the early nineties. I encountered someone who had the capacity to read my heart and be unconditional with my fears and foibles. He was a pioneer and advocate for ending domestic violence and ways to assist male perpetrators to transform their lives. This first significant love relationship introduced me to the world of co-counselling and true partnership. Those short years of our relationship, I experienced being truly loved and supported by a black man. After a few years I became intolerant of the effect of his womanising, on both his own and my Children. My standing as a feminist and public person became insecure, due to his open Polygamy. I felt powerful enough to take a political stance and end my partnership with him. We remain in love as friends to this day. Prior to this experience I had made several mistakes when choosing relationships. In my naivety I had allowed myself to be chosen but had not fully assessed my own choices for being in relationship with others, including my former husband and the father of my lagniappe child. I came to realise that I had also chosen men who were not fully available. This was obviously a reflection of not realising the deep impact of the loss of my father at an early age.

My friendship with A. who passed in 2016, was deeper than I had imagined even though we had been separated for five years before his passing. He has gone to a place where he is no longer in pain, and he will have the peace that he had spoken of many times. I had previously interpreted his need for peace as a way of wanting to shut me up, in other words don't complain or challenge him about what I needed from him that was missing in our friendship. He was significant in his own quiet way because he stayed beside me.

This morning, I woke up with my eyes wet as though I had been crying in my dreams. It's been two days now since he departed, I have taken his name off my contacts list, in case I call him by accident, but I will still speak to him in my mind now that he is further away from the earth. He has become an angel and an ancestor, and I will always remember him as one of my best friends. I got through that loss by re-presenting an image of him on canvas. In a way it keeps him with me as a reminder of his presence in my life. When I look up and see the image on my wall in Tobago, I see that I gave him wings, yet his presence sitting under a Weeping Willow in an open space in England remains with me. Thank you for Sharing part of your life with me. How does one return from the human jungle, when there is no one at home to wash my back, feed me and support my home life.

Kent: August 2019

Saturday morning I'm up early and I'm taking a walk and going to the ocean to clear my mind after attending a workshop. I'm feeling quite sick with the impact of racism. I've used the term 'oppression overload' to describe this experience. Common terms for this state are 'battle fatigue' and 'compassion overload'. This condition arises from long term exposure to oppressions and negativity. Individuals who stand up to the challenges that racism presents, are prone to this. It is a form of trauma that goes with the territory.

I have been doing training. That is what I'm good at. The training has a price because I use an approach which offers compassionate and transformational learning. I feel as though I'm going to die. I think I'm traumatised by the material that I'm working with, and I prepare for what might occur because of the trauma. I survived this week's training about The Challenge of Racism in Therapeutic Practice. BPOC and women attended the seminar, and I am a black woman. There is a cost. I need to recover each time and fully balance my energy again. I don't want to read about racism, and I don't want to hear about it. I want to get back into my cocoon, quietly numbing the pain and freeing myself from this negative energy. I realise a part of me dies every time I lead this training. Then I recover and I reclaim my energy.

As I walk beside the ocean, waves gently roll below, and the gulls sing out their morning melodies. I discovered a Labyrinth in a place that I've never seen before. I wonder whether it appeared for me, or whether I had discovered it. I read the information which suggests that I pause before I enter. I consider a thought. Then I enter and ponder on my wish to create more space in my life for my writing.

This morning, I had an invitation to fill Monday with something. I almost accepted the invitation. As I walk round the circle of the Labyrinth I realise when I reach the centre, that I am the centre of my creativity and it's down to me if I want to make this space. Only I can do it.

Two Tiny white girls on scooters pause to watch me as I exit the labyrinth. One of them asked me 'what's your name?' I tell her my name and I ask her name. I could not pronounce it. It was something like Sherry Anna. She asked me what am I doing? What's that circle? and I tell her it's a Labyrinth. She repeats the word after me several times until she's got it. Her sister, a little shy and a few yards behind her, says nothing. Then two white women, I guess it's their mothers walk past me as if I don't exist. I wanted to say 'good morning' to them and tell them that the little girls learnt a new word this morning, but they are deep in conversation looking straight ahead. I feel silenced. They don't see me, but I am delighted with my new momentary connections. I notice this because it is different from my experience in Tobago, where people passing address each other with a 'good morning' or 'good evening'. The children are not colour blind. They see me. They engage with me, innocently, as an ordinary human.

2023 At a meeting with some of the facilitators trained by me, they asked these questions and commented on the black Empathic Approach to Psychotherapy.

LP.   What is the relationship between a black Empathic Approach and the 'Person-Centred' approach?
LM.   How can two white people display a black Empathic Approach?
UT.   If this is a long-term approach due to repeated racism, how can I help?
RS.   How can I support a black client who just wants to keep their head down?
LP.   It is isolating when you are trying to make your parents proud.
RS.   That is the work, naming the polarities rather than counselling and not noticing an opportunity to build an alliance.

We watched some training videos of vignettes about working with diversity. There were two videos we frequently used to assist participants to observe and discuss the use of a black Empathic Approach. My reflections on the responses demonstrate unravelling of the silence, in therapeutic encounters, that can create colour blindness.

The first is a vignette of a white woman counselling another white woman. The client was portraying unconscious racism. She was quite adamant that having a new, black headmistress, who was changing the school culture of not portraying images and resources that included black people, was in the wrong. We also picked up on the client's intersecting internalised sexism, as she seemed to compare the new black headmistress with the way she followed the instructions of the former white male headmaster. The counsellor, whilst supporting her difficulties, brought her round to realising that she was portraying racist defences towards her colleague.

We also used a vignette portraying the internalised racism of a black woman being presented to a black counsellor. The client was unaware that she was experiencing internalised racism. She spoke of early hurts about her identity, experienced from within the family, namely her skin complexion, the shape of her nose and her hair. She had also experienced unfamiliar feelings when moving from the country area, where she was one of few people of colour, to living in Brixton, where there is a large BPOC community. We examined the dynamic of 'shadism' and 'internalised racism' within the counselling relationship. This was directly related to the use of a black Empathic Approach.

In one of the videos, a white man counselling a black man missed the bits where he spoke directly about the racism he was experiencing. It was helpful to discuss the process in terms of whether a black Empathic Approach had been used. The counsellor was paraphrasing and doing his best to connect, but he failed to use a black Empathic Approach. Applying this approach would have meant that the racism was directly acknowledged in the context of the rage and hurt the client was experiencing. This may also have meant an opportunity for the white councillor to acknowledge their diversity in the context of the subject being presented.

In another vignette a white counsellor, in an attempt to empathise with a black Muslim woman, says that 'he is feeling her pain'. He attempts to address her situation, 'living here', but fails to acknowledge the depth of pain about cultural diversity and racism expressed by this client, though visible, by the tears streaming down her face. There is an obvious lack of attention to deeper feelings expressed by this black woman, due to stereotyping of the strong black woman demeanour. His congruence and ability to demonstrate the compassion needed for a black Empathic Approach to psychotherapy are questionable.

Accepting and applying this concept requires a greater understanding of the self in relation to experiences and the trauma of racism. To develop robustness in this area, therapists need to break through colour blindness and pay full attention to how racialized identity intertwines in the relational dynamics of therapeutic relationships. Analysing the video material in terms of a black Empathic Approach was a useful learning tool. We are left with the question. How do we support individuals in questioning their traditional learning and holding genuine concerns about developing or changing what practices they have become used to?

Colour blindness in the context of racism is a way of dismissing that our diversity exists. I've heard people say, 'I don't see colour', 'we are all the same', 'we are all human and there is one race'. But anti-black racism has caused us to be racialised and colour coded based on whiteness and a range of dark skins.

Hassan (1999) The history of this categorising seems timeless because it goes on. The famous speech purported by Willie Lynch Ref James River in Virginia in 1712 regarding control of slaves within the colony. That, in recent years, has been widely exposed as a hoax. This speech was obviously presented by persons, provoking a system true to this day. Willie Lynch: LET'S MAKE A SLAVE: In my bag here, I HAVE A FULL PROOF METHOD FOR CONTROLLING YOUR BLACK SLAVES. I guarantee every one of you that, if installed correctly, IT WILL CONTROL THE SLAVES FOR AT LEAST 300 HUNDRED YEARS. My method is simple. Any member of your family or your overseer can use it. I HAVE OUTLINED A NUMBER OF DIFFERENCES AMONG THE SLAVES; AND I TAKE THESE DIFFERENCES AND MAKE THEM BIGGER. I USE FEAR, DISTRUST AND ENVY FOR CONTROL PURPOSES. On top of my list is 'AGE', but it's there only because it starts with an 'a'. The second is 'COLOR' or shade. There is INTELLIGENCE, SIZE, SEX, SIZES OF PLANTATIONS, STATUS on plantations, ATTITUDE of owners, whether the slaves live in the valley, on a hill, East, West, North, South, have fine hair, course hair, or is tall or short. Now that you have a list of differences, I shall give you an outline of action, but before that, I shall assure you that DISTRUST IS STRONGER THAN TRUST AND ENVY STRONGER THAN ADULATION, RESPECT OR ADMIRATION

Don't forget, you must pitch the OLD black male vs. the YOUNG black male, and the YOUNG black male against the OLD black male. You must use the DARK skin slaves vs. the LIGHT skin slaves, and the LIGHT skin slaves vs. the DARK skin slaves. You must use the FEMALE vs. the MALE, and the MALE vs. the FEMALE. You must also have white servants and overseers [who] distrust all Blacks. But it is NECESSARY THAT YOUR SLAVES TRUST AND DEPEND ON US. THEY MUST LOVE, RESPECT AND TRUST ONLY US. Gentlemen, these kits are your keys to control. Use them. —IF USED INTENSELY FOR ONE YEAR, THE SLAVES THEMSELVES WILL REMAIN PERPETUALLY DISTRUSTFUL. Thank you, gentlemen.

Colour blindness plays a part in denial of racism and once we acknowledge that racism exists, it becomes more difficult to ignore that we are all unique, special and different, and that skin colour and skin tone cannot be separated from this. In a utopian world, this approach would be ideal, but the damage has been done and our minds have been set to perform differently because of anti-black racism.

A colour-blind approach cannot be justified. We cannot say that men are the same as women and that your disability is the same as mine. We cannot say that camels are the same as pigs. They are all animals, and we are all humans, and history, heritage, and DNA has made us different because of inherent flaws transferred generationally due to an anti-black mindset that separates and undermines humanness.

Having said this I must acknowledge that throughout my career and as a matter of my own CPD, I have become acutely aware of how my light brown skin can affect darker skinned people and white people. This is an area barely touched on between black people and a deficit in attending to therapeutic progress. A BEAP approach does not collude with colour blindness, it helps to break down these defences so that we can lean into the impact of racism rather than avoid it.

Through attending a supervision group that encouraged transparency, Anne, whose voice I presented at the beginning of this chapter, recognised the importance of reflecting on her whiteness and how this created important areas of denial in her development process and therefore colour blindness in her work with black clients. In addressing her previous colour-blindness, she was able to view more clearly intersectional and intergenerational influences on her attitude to others.

This kind of colour blindness can start with disbelief that the oppression of anti-black racism exists. Many people live their lives as colour-blind and blind to the existence of other oppressions. A choice not to see or not to believe and therefore not to witness the experience at the receiving end of anti-black racism is personal. This also contributes to the lack of celebration of BPOC identities. Whether this be ignorance, denial, or unconscious ways of self-protection from engaging with the experience. It does not make the experience unreal. We must ask ourselves whether a decision not to engage with these experiences is useful.

I'm feeling blocked at this point. What is it that I want to say that remains unspeakable today? It kind of feels like there's nothing more to say about this approach but that's absolutely not true. There is a lot to say, and I feel numb. I know my writer's block is temporary and I do feel it's important to write it into the page and try and find out what's there that doesn't want to come out. So, I'm being my own therapist today. I'm trying to kid myself that it's ok to write short chapters. Then I think about what a short chapter is and what is a long chapter. Am I trying to fit into some binary conditioning about how this book should form. Is it my internalised racism shutting me down?

Giving myself the freedom to have a paragraph as a chapter, or ten paragraphs in a chapter is my business. I am in the process of trademarking this concept and I am facing resistance. This refusal has had a profound effect on me. I am up against systemized exclusion, and I can't fit into the criteria for acceptance. I feel small and unintelligent, marginalised and incomplete.

This is a golden opportunity for me to place aside my compulsive independence and ask for help. Something that I have found difficult in my life, and I am now, giving myself permission to do. Sometimes I am quite incongruent about asking for help. I know there's a lot of kindness in the world and I have experienced a lot of kind gestures towards me, yet I have harboured an inner fear of asking for help. I can change this feature, that has long been a coping skill.

I decided to ask two of my closest friends and sister writers to meet with me and help me prepare my warrior self and challenge the office of intellectual property. I feel blessed to have individuals who believe in me and respond when I ask for support. Beneath my confusion and feelings of weakness, about this knock back, there is rage. The rage of being abandoned in my early life, the rage of losing family upbringing and close connections. Now I am enraged by a system that takes my money and locks me out of the recognition I deserve. This rejection came as a message to reinforce my self-compassion and remember my self-care and that validation of this approach is in the book. I foolishly believed that I needed to secure protection for this concept and that British law would assist me to register its use and protect its exploitation. I now relinquish and learn to trust there are higher powers taking care of this project.

My journey of acknowledging compassion for self begins here. Gilbert (2013) claims that compassion helps to soothe distressing emotions and increases feelings of contentment and well-being. (P24) 'The more we understand the way some of our lives are scripted by inner archetypes and mentalities the more we can begin to stand back, take control of them and develop those we choose to develop'. (P28).

> Compassionate behaviour means turning off the angry or sad brain, standing up to some of our own desires and refusing to act on some of our lusts or fears. It can also mean recognising that our intense desire for belonging and connectedness, to be one with a tribe, and defend our own interests can be the source of intense cruelty and atrocity. The tough issue in compassionate behaviour is addressing our own inner tendency towards cruelty.

Summary

In highlighting colour-blindness as a feature of denial in response to anti-black racism, I have shown the need to break through the silences that keep racism in place.

In the next chapter, I discuss the context of empathy as it has been traditionally used, and the possibility of enhancing it as a tool for supporting individuals to emerge from the trauma of anti-black racism and its intersecting oppressions. Namely coming out of colour blindness and using the specific tool of a black Empathic Approach to therapy.

Chapter 2

The context and quality of empathy

Consciously practising empathy requires us to see and hear the other person and take courage to acknowledge what we see and hear through interaction and dialogue. This is a way of checking out the truth about experiences and connecting with feelings. As an adult, I received empathy in a variety of different ways. From family reunions, from friends, in my therapy, and occasionally from colleagues. To make the transition from generic empathy to a black Empathic Approach takes courage and a willingness to interrogate the often taken for granted use of empathy.

Rogers (1959) in Clark Ed (2023. P11) spoke of empathy, as

> the ability to understand another person's experience in the world, perceiving the internal frame of reference of another with accuracy and with the emotional components and meanings which pertain thereto as if you were that person, without ever losing the 'as if' sense. For the time being you lay aside the views and values you hold for yourself in order to enter another's world without prejudice.

It is a way of being with and alongside another person's experience. However, I question whether this is entirely possible in terms of cultural differences and the ways that anti-black racism has permeated the psyche. How do relational practitioners overcome the fears that racism and diversity engender and face the challenge of addressing the elephant in the room.

Individuals are programmed by cultural norms that either integrate or separate us from others, deemed to be privileged or less than worthy of equal respect and loving care. This programming depends on intergenerational, transgenerational community ethics and institutional codes of practice that include family, friendships colleagueship, education, and ways of being.

Many of us are tuned in to oppressive stances either as the oppressor or subject of oppression. We are prone to be in the oppressor group if we have not emerged from the hurt of our experiences of being oppressed. Our defences and ability to empathise are likely to be conditioned by these experiences and ways of coping.

DOI: 10.4324/9781003479994-3

Some unconsciously use code switching (The use of language that fits in with the group or culture we are associating with, to be accepted.) Silencing ourselves, hiding behaviours and self-medication have also become ways of coping with the impact that racism can have on us. I question the depth of empathy of anyone who has been unconsciously in the perpetrator, white privilege group, or who has internalised racism and benefited from this position. Therapists must challenge themselves to unpack the rigid use of traditional theories and expand their use to support cultural identity and the pain of under-managed oppressions such as anti-black racism, in non-defensive ways. Rogers alludes to the benefits of 'metaphor and pace' when listening to others in the counselling setting. If we know that a client's metaphor suggests the pain of racism, do we feel able to expand on that metaphor?

Clark (2023. P13) cites a consensus on a definition of Empathy in Counselling and Psychotherapy. 'Point 10. An empathic capacity to understand a client from multiple ways of knowing'. Clark P15. 'In Rogers view, subjective processing can be emotionally compromised by a practitioner's biases and prejudices leading to distortions in the client's understanding and strains in the therapeutic relationship'. This can happen when denial of racism is present.

Clark (P15) suggests that 'Subjective empathy enables a practitioner to vicariously experience what it is like to be a client for a momentary period of time'. My challenge to this context is that, historically Eurocentric therapy training has not enabled the subjectivity of anti-black racist wounding to be part of training. P16. 'Objective empathy draws from theoretically informed data, credible scholarship, and the accumulated therapeutic experience of a counsellor or therapist in the service of empathically understanding a client'.

Collecting theoretically informed data that impresses ways to transform clients historically, daily and intersectionally wounded by anti-black racism is an essential element of transforming a black Empathic Approach. Clark cites 2010a, Clark & Butler (2020) suggesting that integral empathy in counselling and psychotherapy is consistent with a multiple perspective framework. (Achievement with the feelings and meanings of an individual through the engagement of subjective, objective, and interpersonal modalities.) This view offers some leeway for considering context and systemic influences on levels of empathy and the therapists' level of exposure to antiracist practice.

There are different types of empathy to consider in this discussion. 'Cognitive empathy' is influenced by thought rather than feeling. Questioning this approach can be useful, by locating our inner reconciliation with the impact of racism. We need to ask ourselves whether we can check thoughts influenced by racialisation. Can this work if the supporter is purposefully trying to say the right thing or be politically correct? For example, using the words, 'I hear you' or 'I understand you', or aligning racism with other oppressions, can give the appearance of support, but may not genuinely connect with the other person's feelings and experience.

First, we need to accept that anti-black racism is systemic. It therefore features in everyone's psychological predisposition, whether they are aware of it and accept it or not. Secondly, we need to unpick learned ways of coping with anti-black racism, such as silence and denial. This primary level of self-awareness can lay the foundation for listening and responding to experiences of racism, whether they be articulated or not.

Observing how elephants and giraffes naturally surround each other when their young enter the world, gives us a clue of the naturalness of empathic support in the animal kingdom. Humans are also equipped with this natural empathy for pain, fragility and transformation. We are protective and concerned for our young. How we use our inherited ways of protecting and supporting, become influenced by life experience and education. Collective societies are usually more observant, pro-active and protective of lineage and tribe members. Their empathic responses are usually proactive and conforming. In Western industrial societies, the focus is less on individual well-being and natural ability to demonstrate, and empathy becomes tarnished by the rush for production and economic security.

Our emotional empathy is usually rooted in early genuine connections between ourselves and others and vice versa. Children are naturally empathic with each other and adults, unless they have been severely traumatised and exist in fear and frozen ability to function and get their needs met. They cry together without permission. They connect feelings with experiences and openly express them, until they are shut down. Adultism is one of the earliest oppressions that humans experience from a young age. The ability to experience real connection with feelings and experiences is something we carry into helping roles, unless we have experienced unregulated trauma or self-medicated with drugs and alcohol and are unable to develop natural emotional protection and self-care.

I use the term emotional overload when someone has a build-up of their personal distress and gets tipped over when they listen to another's harsh experiences, concerns, traumas, and tragedies. This can sometimes get converted into what I call the campaigner. (Someone who is supportive of the cause and wants to join the cause or act with, or on behalf of the client's personal story.) This response can be sympathetic rather than empathic and create a level of disconnection and discombobulation, causing the therapists or supporters to be attending to their own needs (role reversal) rather than those of the client. In other words, ejecting themselves out of the counsellor role and into the role of helper and needing help themselves (the counsellor becomes a client). This can be a distraction from connecting with the emotional context of a situation and cause the client to be concerned about the counsellor, as if they have switched roles.

In my own life I am acutely aware, when I am sharing an experience, and the other person responds by talking about their own experience, or something completely different they just want to get off their chest. When this happens, I feel the disconnection and lack of listening. Compassionate empathy is when we feel the pain of another and have the ability to stick with it and convey an appropriate level of acceptance and knowing about the situation, without tipping into our own problems and need for support. These distractions can interfere with listening eyes and heart. They turn attentive listening into intellectual responses. Being mindful of focusing and refocusing on the other person's story is essential to compassionate empathy. Alleyne (2022. P221) 'There are very few references to compassion in situations when coping with racism. Increased compassion can enable easier access to others suffering and pain particularly in the mental and psychological health professions when racism is apparent'.

Making an emotional connection with the other person means you are listening, hearing, understanding, and accepting the associated feelings. It takes time to process emotions in the relational dynamic and this requires trust, patience, compassion without guilt and good attention. It is not about agreeing. It is about creating emotional space by putting aside your own agenda and conveying your connection with the other person's emotions. It is not necessarily about how you word your response but can be portrayed in body language. Reflecting and clarifying can support the connection. This requires self-awareness and self-control. Whether you're listening skills are influenced by psychodynamic, humanistic, or behavioural learning, empathy requires genuineness and courage to go to the place of joy or pain with another person.

Marie was one of the big girls in the children's home for Jews where I was raised. She was a Kindertransport child refugee, who like me had been disconnected from her family of origin. She would have been about 10 years older than me. She was the only person that I remained in contact with after leaving the children's home. I believe our strong connection was deeply embedded in a kind of circumstantial empathy, having both lost our Jewish heritages and family links. One day she told me that when I was a toddler, I used to follow her around as though she were my mother. She said to me "you wanted your mum"' I felt churned up. A mixture of loving connection and gratitude. Drawing on her childhood connection with me, she could see me and empathised with my needs as a child when she was just a teenager. I remember feeling choked up and in a matter of seconds, reliving disconnection, and lack of acknowledgement that I had existed in my own lost world of separation from parents and siblings and lost opportunities of someone touching my heart in that deep intimate connection and knowing. At that moment I knew that someone in the world had connected with my need to belong. At the time I was unaware that there was a term for this kind of connection. Years later when I trained as a counsellor, I began to understand that there is a moment in conversation or counselling when you know you are being heard and seen, lovingly in the context of your life situation. It may even be true that I lived through my teenage years and some of my young adulthood without a deep realisation of this possibility.

A few years ago, I had an opportunity to tour the Nazi work camps in Auschwitz and Birkenau. This tour affected me in a similar way to my experience in Ghana at the slave castles. Inside Elmina Castle I broke down, when I experienced a deeply profound empathic connection with my enslaved African sisters and brothers.

In the empty Nazi workcamps, it was educational for me in that I learned that it was not all Germans, it was those who joined the Nazis who annihilated the Jews. Until then I had internalised a prejudice about Germans. I also learned that anyone deemed to be non-Arian, or imperfectly formed humans, such as black, gay, disabled or even pregnant and not fit for the work of serving the third Reich, and persecution regime, was sent to the gas chambers. I learned that the subjects of this regime were cleansed and shaven prior to being bundled into the gas chambers. I saw the remnants of human bones ground into the earth surrounding the incinerators. I saw the remains of their hair and meagre personal belongings, such as shoes, toothbrushes, false teeth brought with them when they were driven out of their homes. All on show behind glass cabinets. There were thousands of photos of missing individuals of all ages, staring out at a terrifying void and at me as a spectator. I trawled across the images searching for an image of one or two of my lost relatives. Maybe a Hartz, or Wolf, who were never heard of again.

At a later time of practising what I had learned as a counsellor, I sought support for being in a role as a black woman in a world of white privilege. Throughout my training I sought connection through literature created by people who looked like me. I joined a meeting with black counsellors. Joyce, a Jamaican woman responsible for joint authorship of Issues of Race and Culture in counselling Lago, C, and Thompson, J (1991) was at the meeting. Joyce told me there was something that she had noticed about me. Something about the way I held my head on one side and looked sad. Until that moment I had not experienced anyone reflecting that deep level of empathy, associated with body language. Joyce was correct. Her empathy was accurate. I was sad for a long time in my life, and she had taken courage to reflect on what she had seen (I call this an appropriate gaze). I believe that until that point others had only seen my anger. The empathic comment from Joyce and knowing she had taken courage to bring that to my attention was liberating. I took this knowing that I could be heard and understood in terms of the wholeness of my experience as a black woman, therapist, counsellor and trainer into my teaching. Along with my blended identities, I felt a new confidence that my strength and resilience was inherited from ancestral survival and guidance. I am aware that when my feelings are triggered, my whole self is alive with the cultural and relational aspects of my inherited black, Jewish mixed identity, but I give allowance to the fact that my skin colour attracts white racism and internalised racism from both white and BPOC groups.

When I first started presenting 'black Issues workshops' (Later called 'The Challenge of Racism') via BAATN (Black African and Asian Therapist's Network), my work using a Black Empathic Approach was validated. On one occasion a young man came up to me after a workshop and asked if he could personally support my work. We became friends, in fact the first genuine platonic relationship with a black man. P. has supported many workshops actively showing me ongoing support in my life. On one occasion I was harassed by a young white man who lived in the flat underneath me. The police were often on the premises due to his violence to his partner. He presented himself in a thuggish, threatening way, which meant I had to talk to the police about his threatening behaviour. My childhood experiences of being bullied by white boys, in the children's home and knowledge of his racism were triggered and I felt angry and scared. We ended up at a court hearing and P. offered to come to the court and support me and my partner.

Using his own experiences of overt white racism to empathise, he stood beside me and supported us throughout the hearing. I experienced this as an active black Empathic Approach. An ability to notice when this approach is active, assists the ability to practise on a deeper level as a therapist. When you know someone has got your back, the stress of racism is lessened. We lost the case, and my neighbour was let off with a restraining order. He continued to harass me on the street and then things went quiet. After that incident my partner and I were diagnosed with hypertension. The body has its own way of trying to defend itself from physical and emotional attack.

If examined in the context of responding to experiences of anti-black racism, therapists and supporters can use CPD forums to reflect on their own responses to racism. This is not just about being 'woke'. Learning about self and personal responses and coping mechanisms in this context requires individuals to assess their own mindset and learned ways of coping with everyday racism, and institutional racism.

Becoming an expert at creating safe holding dialogue about this oppression, includes taking a risk to address both covert and overt experiences of racism. In addition, intersectional experiences that merge with racism need to be considered. This may seem like a huge additional task. Thoughts about focussing on ways to emerge from the traumatic impact of racism are a valuable resource for progress into an evolved sense of practice where gradually a black Empathic Approach becomes natural.

This process of monitoring is paramount when harnessing a black Empathic Approach as a skill set in the helping professions. It is not just a switching on, or a transfer of empathy, it requires self-acceptance, patience and a relationship with racism and the powerful feelings associated with anti-black racism (recognition trauma). Attending a variety of emotional responses such as denial, silence, guilt, and rage, associated with the trauma that racism can cause is a vital component in developing a black Empathic Approach to therapy.

Secondary defences can show up if we try and avoid working through the process of attending to racism. For people of colour, code switching, hypervigilance and low self-esteem can occur. Chronic diseases brought on by continuous distress, overwork and low self-esteem can be exacerbated. Behaviours that arise because of internalising racism often go unnoticed and therefore unattended.

My experience is that white people expose fragility and defend with silence, resulting in subjects of racism feeling responsible for their plight and that they cannot name or question their experiences in the presence of perpetrators. Eddoe

Lodge (2018) conveyed her experiences of empathy lack. I connect with her despair when she talks about the difficulty that white people have when BPOC individuals want to share an experience of racism. The empathy she received was mainly from BPOC, who like her, had experienced similar.

Of course, there was a backlash and a book called 'Why I'm no longer talking to black people about Race & George Floyd' Gemmel (2020) has publicly perpetrated, rather than empathised, because he can. It is non-empathic and blaming. In defence of his whiteness, he feels it is ok to put forward a generalised explanation of what racism is. He diagnosed black people with an 'oppression complex' using black on black murders, fatherless children and subnormal education as a backdrop to this conditioned response rather than institutional racism. Then he cites Obama, obtaining world power as an example of achieving aspirations and a contradiction to the oppression complex. In his tiny mind, he wants us to believe that racial profiling does not exist. He claims that the killings of George Floyd, Brianna Taylor, and Michael Brown were 'nonracist', citing police brutality over racism, due to the ethnicity of the police. This kind of push back, commanding attention to a distorted form of white fragility, disgusts me. It is not empathic, and it is the epitome of gaslighting and white racism. He wants us to believe that we are socialised into a victim mindset and accuses black people of fuelling racism with an 'oppression complex'. From the perspective of a US white man, he is intellectualising and disrespecting Eddoe Lodge's reference points. This kind of thinking can lead to the subjects of racism questioning their own mental health. I feel deeply disturbed that anyone in their right mind would seek to undermine the stories of BPOC experience. He uses his entitlement and privilege to judge and assume that this is ok.

Copenhagen 2023

I am in a Jewish Museum in Proviantpassagen 6 watching 3d images about Danish and Polish Jews fleeing from their homes, like my Grandparents, during the pogroms. Many fled to Sweden in boats and were treated as unwelcome strangers. It is hard to imagine the levels of distress that they would have felt, leaving their life belongings and taking the barest of essentials with them. On display there were explanations of some of the challenges of settling and agreeing, between themselves rules for continuing their faith and supporting each other. The floors in the Museum are slanted at different angles, giving the effect of being on a boat. I am told, this mirrors the experience of the fleeing immigrants. It made me feel queasy and I had to sit and recover. I am realising how sharp my senses are. My body is easily interrupted by smells, tastes and movement and I am happy to be alive and affected by the environment. On reflection, I tell myself that I am more deeply connected to my Jewish ancestral heritage, than I am aware of.

In considering the varied views and approaches to empathy I believe that combining a subjective and objective stance using an integral model that incorporates both 'emic' and 'ethic' considerations in the use of cultural nuances and in considering cultural assumptions, may be useful for the development of a black Empathic Approach. Clark (2022. P35)

> Objective empathy involves going beyond merely calculating and evaluating items from a self-report personality inventory or completing a rote scanning of a behavioural checklist to categorise the psychopathology of a client. Instead, a practitioner assumes an empathic position by reflecting on how objectively derived findings illuminate what life is like for an individual in lived context.

In a subjective integration with this approach, the client's lived experience of racism and consideration of the therapist's attitude and way of being, combined with their alignment to systemic power that perpetuates racism, is important. This would allow for consideration of the client's daily struggles and the nature of the client's cultural and racialised background and coping mechanisms in this area.

Summary

Attempting to transform empathy can be a challenging prospect, because of this being a therapeutic approach that may be taken for granted. I have shown how reflecting on my own experiences and growing compassion has influenced a way that empathy can be transformed for use as an antiracist tool. As explained, there are different dimensions to a black Empathic Approach, and therefore viewing empathy holistically from the subject's experience and perpetrator context is important. In the first instance therapists should be willing to lean into the antiracist experience and consider their responses to anti-black racism.

Chapter 3

Breathing new life into empathy

I was separated from my biological family at the age of five months and had no choice about where I was raised. I experienced a powerful white gaze from carers at an early age, growing up in a predominantly white children's home in South London with no adult BPOC models present. No dialogue about my isolated situation as the only child of colour, and the loss of parental closeness was offered. Absence of this bonding was ignored, and I was fed, watered, clothed and raised in ignorance of this gap in my identity development. This was my norm, and I do not have a memory of being consciously aware of what was missing, in terms of affirmation and my identity. I discovered my skin colour when it was pointed out by other children.

As a teenager I was often blamed for my behaviour rather than supportively coached into transforming delinquent ways of getting my needs met. Being parentless, there was little in me to trust the projections that I was subject to as a young black girl. In truth, I was silenced. I became an expert at selective mutation and withdrew inside myself for protection. Unknowingly, I was a warrior standing on the shoulders of my ancestors. I developed a sense of righteous indignation that helped me to support myself. This is not an ideal situation for a child, but because of these experiences, I became fiercely independent and developed an inner voice about justice. I guess that is one of my strengths now.

It would be easy to say I am naturally empathic to the pain of others. I am kind, I am an attentive listener, I understand the place of empathy in therapeutic contexts because I am well practised at connecting through my heart with others and walking alongside them. So why would I need to do anything other than what I'm doing now?

Therapists, clients and caregivers exposed either directly or vicariously to the trauma of racism, experience a range of powerful related feelings. I named these powerful feelings 'recognition trauma'. This can feel like emerging from sinking sand and disbelief that we have it in us to approach this theme with confidence. The theme of recognition of trauma is associated with the impact of racism and other intersecting oppressions, and the coping skills we often use to keep safe from further trauma and retraumatisation. This approach requires the development

DOI: 10.4324/9781003479994-4

of what I have called an 'appropriate gaze'. I will elaborate on this concept in Chapter 7.

UK 2023

I'm sitting in a white space listening to black music and writing about empathy. The waiters smile sweetly at me as they serve vegan food and what I call healthy coffee. I ponder on how the production of vegan food and healthy dietary requirements have caught on within a few years, but attitudes to connecting in healthy ways with people of colour are so very slow in changing.

I'm feeling blocked at this point. What is it that I want to say that remains unspeakable today? It kind of feels like there's nothing more to say about this approach, but that's absolutely not true. There is a lot to say, and I feel numb. I know this writer's block is temporary and I do feel it's important to write it into the page and try and find out what's there that doesn't want to come out. I'm being my own therapist today. I'm trying to kid myself that it's ok to write short chapters. Then I think, what is a short chapter? What is a long chapter? Am I trying to fit into some binary conditioning about how this book should form? Giving myself the freedom to have a paragraph as a chapter, or ten paragraphs in a chapter is my business.

I am in the process of trademarking the concept of a 'black Empathic Approach' and I am facing resistance. This is a golden opportunity for me to ask for help. Something that I have found difficult in my life, and I am now, giving myself permission to do. Sometimes I am quite incongruent about asking for help. I know there's a lot of kindness in the world and I have experienced a lot of kind gestures towards me, yet I have harboured an inner fear of asking for help. I jump the fear cavern and ask two of my closest friends and sister writers to meet with me and help me prepare my warrior self to challenge the Office of Intellectual Property. If it wasn't for them, I would have given up at that point.

My research started with the title 'Black Issues'. Taking into account diversity, and many dimensions of this concept, whilst not dashing the baby away with the bath water. Last night I dreamed about a baby that I was frantically trying to prepare to feed. I came round to wondering if that baby was me because I often feel starved of nurturing and validation as a person of colour, and as a human being with a parallel life running alongside this legacy work.

I realise that in my personal life, I rarely talk to others about my work of supporting and healing the trauma of racism. The reason for this is that I fear and expect humiliation, because I appear confident and clear about the pain of racism and often this is an unspeakable area for others. Correcting this lack of safety is fundamental to a black Empathic Approach to therapy. I wanted an opportunity to dialogue and open a space for mutual healing in this area, but sometimes I hurt because my expectations are not fulfilled. Then I go into hiding to keep my mental health safe. Writing it out in this book is a way of self-empathising and sharing my own empathic journey with others.

UK 2023

It is early morning, and I am taking a stroll. I feel slow but energised. I reflect on a recent experience with horses. This was the second time attending the 'Equine Experience' at Checkenden farm. An experience led by D, another ex-supervisee. She's accompanied by B, who I met on my first experience with the horses. There were nine of us, eight being people of colour. I attended with the intention of building on my growing confidence about being with big animals. I think big animals represent big scary humans, especially big scary men. This was level two for me. I wanted to build on getting close to these huge animals without fear. When we were in the field, I decided to be still and see what happened. A couple of horses approached me, and I noticed that if I made sudden movements they were startled. This seemed to reflect the fear I was feeling inside. Paying attention to the sensitivity and noticing my own vulnerability gave me clues as to how to be with them. Eventually one horse came very close and nuzzled me and I was able to talk to her and stroke her with less fear than my previous experience. She gave me permission to stroke her mane and her head. Then she turned her head to me, and we had a few moments quietly looking into each other's eyes and acknowledging the calmness and sensitivity of a mutual gaze.

This was a unique experience for me and my second experience of a horse knowing and sensitively connecting to me. There was a quiet empathic connection that I momentarily trusted. There were no words, but something emotional happened, between me and a very different animal. Eventually another horse came and stood quietly close to the one next to me. I was between two large animals who stayed calmly observing me and allowing me to be close, using both my hands to stroke them and notice them sharing their love with me. There was something in the closeness and stillness that evoked a new sense of trust in me. I felt emotional, and that I had broken through a trust barrier about being close to humans, that had been demolished way back in my childhood. Someone who I had been very close to told me once that I frightened people with my fear. I had no idea that I was wearing my fear that loudly. This experience with the horses showed me that if I could tame my own fear, they could get closer. It was clear that they had gained some trust in me, and I felt able to become close. Although I am reflecting on an experience that happened just a few days ago, I am noticing how this has supported my personal development. I have found a way to overcome some of my fears about communicating the real me and when challenges occur, I am telling myself that I am more powerful now and I can be less afraid to connect. Of course, a two-way process must happen for empathy to be appropriately given and received. Just as I had experienced with the horses. I still believe that to help heal the traumatic impact of racism, we need some communication that attends to this specific hurt and the discourses that perpetuate it.

UK 2023

*It is late September I am held up in England, when I should have arrived in Tobago two weeks ago. It is a sunny Friday afternoon. I am in a beach Café with my laptop, feeling relieved at having the time to return to my writing. I've been distracted by organising legacy workshops to promote this approach. I have been writing to publishers and taking care of my health. Only other artists and creators can feel empathy with the way life's distractions take us away from our focus. I spent an hour replying to important emails and figuring out a response to a jargonised refusal from the intellectual property office. Once again, I feel that the term 'black Empathic Approach' is being misunderstood and misinterpreted. A second refusal has made me more determined to fight for this concept, but it must take me a few weeks to gather myself into a calm space where I can think rationally about my response. Now I want to take this to a senior officer to give me a fair chance to understand the meaning of some of the jargon. My immediate response was feeling oppressed by the language. Carl Marx would call this 'specialised knowledge' that maintains class divisions. My oppression in this situation is linked to having grown without the tools to understand intellectualised presentations and vocabularies, whether they be verbal or written. I feel excluded, humiliated and disempowered. I do not possess an extensive vocabulary, if that includes Eurocentric jargon of the middle and upper classes, yet I know I am not stupid. I guess these situations underpin the imposter syndrome. (Imposter syndrome is the condition of feeling anxious and not experiencing success internally, despite being high-performing in external, objective ways. This condition often results in people feeling like 'a fraud' or 'a phony' and doubting their abilities (*www.betterup.com/blog/what-is-impos ter-syndrome-and-how-to-avoid-it*)*

At school, I was good at quoting my times tables, but I never raised my hand to answer general knowledge questions. I felt uninformed and dumb, and no one noticed except me. Consequently no one assisted me with my voiceless experience. A true account of my abandonment and rejection. I carried that feeling inside of me until I had my first short story published. This story was called 'Yearning to belong'. (1988) Someone from a feminist publisher noticed that my experience was important and to be shared. I was shocked that writing something so very personal about my experience was valued. My impostor syndrome has gradually eroded as a postgraduate. Along my journey others have shared similar experiences, either they have shared their problems of understanding theory, or they have said they are dyslexic. The sharing has enabled me to see where I place myself in terms of feeling unintelligent and not academic. I experienced empathy because of our shared feelings and experience.

Not a lot has been written about empathy as a healing tool and in itself a thera-peutic approach that can support anti-black racism. Empathy does not stand alone, but of course, it creates a foundation for healing and mutual communication about trauma and oppression. I have a strong conviction that an explanation of empathy and its use in healing the trauma of personal and systemic racism can assist the development of training, practice and supervision in psychotherapy and counselling. Although the black Empathic Approach may come across as a simplistic term that can be straightforwardly applied, there are complex nuances that need to be taken on board, in terms of self-reflection, personal relationship with empathy and racism and genuine application, rather than just plain empathy.

The approach has been tried and tested with groups of people in therapeutic disciplines and the caring professions. There are times when I have thrown my arms up in despair, because assimilation and coercion of Eurocentric thinking, implanted into training and regular everyday thinking, has caused a smokescreen and complacency. We are enough to offer empathic responses, but we are not all woke enough to engage in a black Empathic Approach.

For this approach, I cannot underestimate the importance of gaining personal knowledge and self-acceptance, combined with the way we internalise and cope with knowledge and experience of racism. What should follow this is enough self-care to know and accept the challenges of using this approach while withstanding the backlash and defensiveness that can arise from being clear when applying it. Sometimes there is an expectation of collusion within the pushback, whether rooted in white fragility or internalised racism. It is important to study, take on board and challenge works that have been presented by white professionals in the field of psychotherapy and counselling, so that they can be recognised as allies. This helps to reinforce the truth about the damage that racism can cause, and the depth of healing needed to clean up its aftermath. The incident of child Q, and the pavement lynching of George Floyd, to name but a few, have clearly demonstrated the vicarious trauma associated with systemized anti-black racism.

Below I present parts of a discussion with facilitators trained in a black Empathic Approach. We have been gathering observations from video counselling sessions representing diversity.

Question from L: How do two white people display the BEA approach?

Dr. Isha: BEA does not have a colour to it, it is about what is in your heart, it is about courage, clarity, congruence and knowing your relationship with racism and racialisation. It is an active decision to work with the trauma of racism. As we know there can be denial and collusion when working with white privilege, experiences of racism in the news, school or with partners and friends. It is about an openness to address that anti-black racism comes from many areas. It is about understanding that people in the perpetrator group have their own recognition trauma and BPOC folks have recognition trauma based on their internalised racism and intersecting oppressions.

There are different levels when two white people are addressing racism. In the video we watched, the white counsellor was trying to address it, and she was doing her best. Some of the participants in the workshop group see this and get angry and accuse the therapist of calling the client racist. When I carried out my doctoral research, the white students were afraid of being called racist, rather than exploring their positioning of white privilege. The therapist in the video did not directly accuse the client of racism, she gently drew it out of the client and was not intending to collude with the client. She knew what was going on. Her approach is softly, and she is doing her best, as training has taught her to go softly, but as observers, we can see the client's denial and her rage.

I would have addressed this by drawing the white client's attention to the Head teacher. 'You are talking about who has placed the images of Black and Asian people on the wall. Why is that an issue for you? Is it their skin colour?' Have you learnt about yourself in relation to the black Headmistress? Do you realise that there is much more information you may need about how you are understanding and reacting to this black head teacher. The client may have got angry, which she does. She asks the therapist, 'are you saying I am racist'? She is also awakening at the same time. It means carving out a BEA to suit the situation. The most important thing is to address it, otherwise, collusive denial takes over.

Question from U- It is upsetting working with someone long term and It's the second time they are leaving the job due to racism. What is it like for you as a black woman? When racism feels so overwhelming and how can BEA approach work when I as a counsellor, in the counter transference feel redundant or overwhelmed, or helpless.

Dr. Isha: What is happening to you? You are internalising something in the counter transference. Then what happens to your therapeutic relationship?

U-   I am internalising something.

Dr. Isha: You have gone out of a counsellor role you need something. Somehow this scenario pushes you off balance. You need to understand we have the knowledge that racism is an everyday experience. It is not something that only happens twice in a job, it has happened before, and it will happen again. Working with this depends on your self-care in terms of working with your internalised racism. You know the areas you get knocked off balance and need self-care. Your client needs to leave their job two times. You need to take it to therapy and supervision each time. If your own therapist or supervisor is not robust enough to offer a black Empathic Approach, you will get worn down, sucked into your own distresses. You may not even be aware that your soul is being gnawed away and your identity becoming less recognizable. This disempowering trait can create havoc for those in the facilitation role.

Alleyne (2022) talks about the trauma and burden of heritage as an enduring cycle of events grinding down the individual persona.

Witnessing this experience can create vicarious trauma in the therapist who may then be at risk of an incongruent gaze.

Question from R- An Islamic woman feels forced out of her job. Because of her financial situation, she wants me to show how she can keep her head down and keep her job. I feel torn, she says she needs to keep her head down and nod, and this reminds me of slavery. I am telling her, it's not her fault; it's the management. She may not be able to receive it,

Dr.Isha -   How would you present this to the client? Can the client receive some BEA?

R –   Maybe I cant rescue, there is something about challenge, how can she hold her head up high under impossible circumstances?

Dr.Isha: Feels heart-breaking – if you are heartbroken, that is the place to go. I once said to my counsellor" I am afraid I am going to breakdown". The therapist said, "Have your breakdown". I am giving you permission to work with your client and her broken heart, that is part of working with BEA. You can explain racism and islamophobia. You can't save her. You cannot advise her. It is heart-breaking to her, and she wants to keep her head down. What is it like as a Muslim woman of colour to keep her head down? Can you see that we can do this? You cannot fix her. No matter what happens you are still in the role of a therapist.

In another vignette we watched a white woman counselling a black man who is clearly feeling demoralised, exasperated and despairing.

L –   The counsellor is doing her best, but she misses the bits on talking about racism. She does not attend to talking about being a black man. She doesn't name racism. She is not with his experience of racism. She does not look comfortable. She just says "how does it make you feel?" When she already knows how painful racism is for this client. What makes her hold back on connecting empathically with this experience.

U –   I feel angry, it's outrageous. The client says, 'I have to leave it and carry on'.

Dr.Isha: She does not appear to be a robust enough counsellor to go into racism. It's no good to feel sorry for him. It does not work with the trauma of racism.

L -   I found the counsellor patronising, it took her ages to address him as a 'black man' and it was a circular session. The client was raising another point. The difference between first- and second-generation experiences of racism. Being expected to do better than our parents in dealing with covert racism. They have done their best, but as first generation. They are under this pressure to do better than their parents.

Dr.Isha: There is a whole intergenerational and transgenerational history that clients carry. We need consideration of racism, migration – trans and inter-generational aspects in our approach. BEA is about being curious about how the family has dealt with racism. i.e. keep my head down and carry on. Internalising all the trauma that goes with the experience of racism and not allowed to be enraged. It is important to unpick where the coping skills were learned. We need to just carry on with learning about racism. i.e. how did you cope at an early age with racism, pre-school etc

Dr.Isha: Remember that nursery children are so called treated the same.

Coat on the hook, all had Christian assembly when I was a child. In secondary school, my peer group – the black girls were shouted at in racist terms. What kind of confusion is that? I am ninety-nine percent sure there is a history and accumulation of trauma around racism. There is a history of the coping skills of racism that comes from how we were raised, what we saw, and whether we had supportive discussions about it or not? The institutes of psychotherapy have let us down. We are working on ourselves and it's important to be gentle.

Dr. Isha: The videos are a good attempt at working with diversity and counselling, before people dared to call it working with racism. Times are changing. The Chief of Scotland Yard, England is saying the institute is racist. Ok -who is he trying to tell that too? Things are moving forward. We have not gone very far but we can name it. The videos we are watching were made when it was not safe to name racism, that is why BEAP is important. We are taking it to pieces to look at how empathy can be shifted and moved forward and transformed into working with the damage that racism has done, there will be a lot of resistance for people who believe that a generic approach is just ok. They may continue denial and continue to hide. Clients need to have their identity valued in terms of the damage that racism and trauma does. With white people it also traumatises and damages them. I am writing about this because, those are areas that are seemingly untouched in the discourses of therapy training.

Dr. Isha: In one video I saw a black woman wearing a hijab. She had tears streaming from her eyes. The counsellor, a white man, is not paying any attention. I noted 'strong black woman'. He was not attending to feelings. He was busy paraphrasing, to the best of his ability, and there did not appear to be a connection. This is a significant response to black women. You don't see the tears; you are not attending to them. It is attended to in a patterned way, that keeps the counsellor outside of his feelings and her shared emotions. He does not appear concerned. It is very painful to watch. Black women are not meant to feel that deeply and often our deep feelings do not get acknowledged because we are not seen as fragile, we are seen to cope. She was sent to him by a tutor. Was he the right counsellor for her? That was not a BEA approach, and I would not show this to a group who are trying to learn about BEAP.

I want to encourage conscious empathy, built around awareness of self in relation to Black issues. Empathy is a multi-disciplinary skill that provides a useful starting point for a transtheoretical approach. A transtheoretical approach considers the use of concepts that can be integrated into a variety of therapeutic models. I shall follow this thread by considering and following empathy and a transcultural focus on black issues. This means, to recognise and understand invisibility. To notice skin colour on the spectrum of racist experience. For example, a person of colour may have their experience marginalised if they are very light skinned. It means engaging with a context of racism that may be apparent, or not necessarily identified by the client. it means that you are working with the context of racism and racialisation even if the client is not addressing it themselves. It is important to find ways to address it, either directly with the client, or in your supervision, and in your peer groups. You are working with it because you are the therapist. Therefore, you are working with the relational process, and you are working with it for the client and with the client. You are becoming clearer on it when you are actually doing the face-to-face work.

A Black Empathic Approach organises and links the experience of internalised imagery and negative imagination and places it in the context of real lives. To achieve this the therapist's early experiences of oppression based on their skin colour, caste and experiences of hair texture, must be processed in the context of his or her exposure to white Western influences. In life and in relationship to the therapist, a client's experience must be taken into account, as in how we feel about each other, as white or BPOC. There is a lot of background work that needs to be done for the therapist to be robust enough. We need to use our wisdom, to approach what we know is obvious, whether the client is saying it, or not. When we consider a black Empathic approach it is important to acknowledge racism is a discourse and culture ingrained within other cultures.

The development of BEAP will help clients to eliminate the need to explain or justify experiences of racism. For black counsellors working with black clients, careful attention needs to be given in creating empathy from shared experiences rather than subjective identification, i.e., the counsellor expressing they have experienced the same, or similar. This allows empathy to be experienced in a deeper context of my BPOC experience and the experience of others. I place an emphasis on facilitating black trainees and black clients to do that work, not just a focus on racism. A focus on our learning and on our development and robustness with both black and white clients in this area. Also, a focus on internalised racism, shadeism/colourism. How we have internalised racism and whether we have processed our own hurts within the colour spectrum and used this knowledge to help others.

Sometimes Eurocentric theory and training get in the way of the black Empathicapproach. During BEA workshops we witness confusion about risking the challenge of this approach that may not have been attended to during therapy training. It is often difficult for students to conceive that there are other ways of being when working with the impact of racism. Eurocentric training has to an extent enslaved our minds and coerced binary approaches that lead us to believe that any other approach could be wrong or damaging for clients.

All this confusion can result in resistance to even trying it out. If we disbelieve in our ability to develop this approach and our freedom to decide ways of emerging from the trauma of racism, we are then at risk of being caught up in a vicious cycle of denial, fear and powerlessness, that can morph into perpetrator behaviour.

Empathy is not something that can be pushed from behind or pulled from in front. It has its own momentum and personal connection to the soul of the giver. If therefore it is personal and not a patterned way of offering support, we are at liberty to mould it into something meaningful, relating to the experience.

In the case of racism, it may not be recognised if the experience is not clearly identified by the therapist or supporter, in a way that connects with the client or receiver's experience. A bit like saying 'I hear you' when someone is describing a problem, rather than clearly stating what they are hearing about the oppression related to skin colour, ethnicity and cultural designation.

Therapists can try this exercise out as a way of finding an appropriate connection with the experience and trauma of racism.

1 Ask someone to describe an experience of racism.
2 Respond by being oblique and saying something like I hear you.
3 Try listening to the experience again and using a response that directly acknowledges the experience of skin colour oppression.
4 Ask the subject of the racism to reflect back to you which response felt more authentic and more connected to the experience of racism.

This simple test can introduce a listener to a functional way of applying a black Empathic Approach. Giving attention and responding to someone who is traumatised by racism involves an 'appropriate gaze' and black empathic listening.

Summary

In this chapter, I shared discussions about observing and developing the practice of a black Empathic Approach. I captured my experience of personal development, that included overcoming fears and reclaiming my power to demand respect by using the concept of a black Empathic Approach. Although not made explicit, I am aware that my rage has fuelled the determination that pushes me forward in promoting a black Empathic Approach.

Chapter 4

Assimilation and humiliation

Tobago 2017

I am seeing how deep humiliation runs for Caribbean people that I am surrounded by daily. I am also beginning to get it. How difficult it must be to shift your life from living in a warm musical climate embraced by tropical elements, to 'the mother country', greeted by a concrete jungle, and the cycle of anti-black racism and biased attitudes towards skin colour, that have filtered through generations. When I am in England, closed in from cold dark winter nights. I understand how sunshine, and laughter play a central part in coping and everyday life for African and Caribbean peoples.

I was born in Birmingham England and became a British citizen by rights of my father holding a colonial passport and my mother whose family were former European citizens, fleeing from the pogroms and terror of the Nazi ethnic cleansing regime. I am a descendent of immigrants, of ethnic cleansing and slavery. The essence of my empathy goes way back before my birth. This history and heritage underpins my concept of a black Empathic Approach. Through research I discovered a letter my father wrote, stating that he and his wife were from the two most hated peoples. My father, a pan Africanist was born in Trinidad and Tobago in 1898. He came to Britain in 1930. Unable to establish work as a writer and teacher, he focused his attention on equality and justice in Africa, the Caribbean and Europe. The middle passage as he knew it. It is possible that his father, being the proprietor of a cocoa plantation, in the Caribbean, was a descendant of freed slaves. As I embark on this book Trinidad and Tobago celebrates 60 years of Independence from colonial power, and assimilation with the British Empire. Although the traits of colonialism are embedded in the attitudes of many indigenous Caribbean peoples, I too embrace my colonial heritage that was not acknowledged at home or in school in the UK. Here is the letter written by my father to the children's home where I was placed in 1949.

Dear sir or Madam,
I visited London last week with the object of calling on you for the purpose of making arrangements for handing over three children of Jewish connection

DOI: 10.4324/9781003479994-5

to you if there be room in your homes. The following are facts my wife is a Jewess, and I am a Negro. The two races are classified as inferior by Hitler and my race is so classified by all other peoples in the world, including the English. Although I have produced a good home wherein, I hoped to bring up my children in accordance with the Christian practice, I find that the home is on the verge of breaking through pressure put on my wife by her family members who are bitterly prejudice against my complexion. My wife declares that she finds it wholly impossible to care for the children, and so I must find somewhere to put them.

I am looking back at this period of my life, where I was ejected from my family home, due to poverty, mental health and anti-black racism and placed in a children's home. The proprietors of the home were white, Ashkenazi Jews converted to missionaries, whose purpose was to convert children of their own people to Christians, so they might be saved from annihilation due to their identities. This was a confused beginning for a young black girl. Being shifted from racism and internalised antisemitism within the family to another institution perpetrating a form of mental ethnic cleansing, to procure assimilation, proposed to keep children safe. I am reminded of a rabbit proof fence story in Australia. The land from indigenous peoples was taken and their children stolen. They were taken into missionary care by Jesuit priests and into a conversion scheme that would breed the melanin out of their skin, in order to whitewash the nation and make those with darker skins more manageable.[1]

The forcible removal of First Nations children from their families was based on *assimilation* policies, which claimed that the lives of First Nations people would be improved if they became part of white society. Assimilation policies proposed that Aboriginal and Torres Strait Islander Peoples should be allowed to 'die out' through a process of natural elimination, or, where possible, assimilated into the white community (Behrendt 2012).

This was an enforced assimilation in the name of religion and Western interference within the communities and cultures of indigenous peoples. On my visit to Perth Australia and visiting cultural museums, I came across stories of 'truth and reconciliation' that were heartbreaking. It was also clear that the consequences of this atrocity in Australian history are still evident within indigenous communities today.

As the daughter of colonised parents, I too am colonised and assimilated. I write through the eyes and resistance of a colonised being. My attempts to be transparent may be highly influenced by my own assimilation and humiliation. I am however convinced that my survival of these two evils, created my rebellious curiosity about transforming the discourse of empathy.

As a result of the Windrush scandal and gaslighting by the home office, the lives of black people from African, Caribbean and some Asian communities in the UK have been fundamentally different from those of white communities. A report from the Home Office Team, reporting on the Windrush scandal, states. 'Major immigration legislation in 1962, 1968 and 1971 was designed to reduce the proportion of people living in the United Kingdom who did not have white skin'. The Guardian Amelia Gentleman

www.theguardian.com › uk-news › may › wind. 29 May 2022.

The report summarises decades of 'dysfunctional relationships between Britain's institutions and black and minority ethnic people', It concludes: 'The politics of Britain's borders, which have been administered for more than a century by the Home Office, are now inextricably connected with race and with Britain's colonial history'. Tony Sewell's Commission on Race and Ethnic Disparities (2021) declared that there was no evidence to suggest that Britain was an institutionally racist place. Then, the prime minister told parliament: 'For centuries, our United Kingdom has had a proud history of welcoming people from overseas'.

Simon Woolley, the former CEO of Operation Black Vote and chair of the No 10 race disparity unit July 2020, said "the refusal to make the report public was shameful. 'The government is hellbent in its denial of the systemic nature of racial inequality and in this climate historical facts have become uncomfortable truths that need to be hidden'. 29 May 2022 17.15 BST Amelia Gentleman, The Guardian.

We did not need another meeting, or another Commission, to inform us that racism is systemic. Who was this Commission for, and whose money was used for this purpose? Saying it on paper does not evidence a thing, or undo the trauma caused by this pervasive discourse. I am heartbroken at the plight of those individuals who were deemed to be illegal by the UK immigration system, after decades of post-war rebuilding and supporting British institutions, including the health service. These efforts inherited from British colonialism were active forms of assimilation, followed by deep humiliation. They were based on trust that the 'mother country' would embrace their efforts to integrate and become part of British society.

My father would have turned in his grave as he, being one of a few immigrants who arrived earlier than the Windrush era on a British colonial passport, supported those arriving during this period. This is assimilation followed by gross humiliation.

Commonwealth citizens left their lives in the Caribbean, under the illusion that they had been invited to better their lives and help build Britain. The humiliation of many lives and families being shattered, contributed to confused regrets about this invitation, followed by rejection, based on accusations of false presentation of their immigration status. This amounts to gaslighting and humiliation. The equivalent of having the rug pulled from under their feet. The issue of declaring non-immigrant status after decades of settling with their families in the UK was absurd, humiliating, and deeply painful.

This scenario of assimilation followed by humiliation underlies grief and mental health in black families across the nation. A response of personal and community outrage rippled across BPOC communities. Empathy for their plight came from community interest and those affected by this awful dilemma. On top of everyday racism and the consequences of losing residential status, family connections and community origins, individuals have suffered ill health, death, repatriation and loss of current and previously relinquished communities. For those who were not directly affected, this traumatic situation underpins a transgenerational process that constitutes an aspect of fundamental grief in BPOC mental health.

The rage that lies beneath this mistreatment has added to unstable mental health and a lack of trust in our communities. Accepting and reaching into the powerful feelings that underpin this experience is a must in the process of a black Empathic Approach and healing process in therapy and mental health support. One of the ways that I manage my rage about personal and institutional racism is by writing poetry.

A poem for my long-lost father: Celebrating the 75th anniversary of the Fifth Pan-African Congress (*Jul 2020)*

POEM DEAR FATHER

(Dr. Isha Mckenzie-Mavinga (2020) Dear Father
(Dedication to Ernest Mckenzie-Mavinga son of freed slaves 1898–1948)

You created me
a micro seed
then left forever
a legacy
to discover

You were there
defending
lives that matter
now more than ever

adrift
from colonised Islands
where tranquil waters flowed
You thought England
resembled back home
except
churches were empty
It was cold

You visioned equality
your contemporaries
strong together
Dubois, Padmore,
Rojas, Appiah
Garvey, Kenyatta,

Nkrumah
Luther King
Obama

against attitudes
impoverished
that don't work
in our favour
they reinforce
adverse behaviour
Racism a pandemic
like any other

You survived
between wars
supported
mother country
pulled out dead
from the debris
raised the game
for your sisters
your brothers
arrival thwarted
barred colours
thorn in the side
of others

your voice found
at Hyde Park Corner
Strong
never empty
weakened
during Conference
by skin bourgeoisie

an educational elitism
played out in history
in the islands
the struggle
was a travesty

Sankofa bird
looked back
on poverty

strife in oil fields
inequality
between
indentured labourers
between
descendants
of enslaved survivors

You visioned onwards
from racial abuse
towards
your blended family
giving not a dam
known around town
the tall Noble looking
coloured gentleman
customary
three-piece suit
doffed your hat
to local chit chat

in a multiple dwelling
one room rented
staved off winter
huddled round
paraffin heater
documented findings
proclaimed future
charity and peace

You compromised
your health
prioritised labour
expired
before a chance
to be my saviour

in spirit your struggle
still alive
evolved, laid bare
once more
as Covid dust settles
the seeds you planted
thrive

grown stronger, taller,
greater, more inspired

hopeful once again
for equality, respect
dignity, humility
that creed and race
find equal place'
in your name
Mavinga

Although
I cannot see you
I know that
you are in me
If only
I could feel you
My choices would
have pleased you
taken all sadness
right away
then I wouldn't
Grieve you
Dear Father

Humiliation runs deep in the lives of many individuals. Most people have been subject to personal or group humiliation. The role of shame and being shamed underlie humiliation. Shame is instilled in humans at an early age. The ways we are disciplined that certain behaviours are wrong or when we are punished because adults believe we might be causing them to feel their own shame. Aspects of shame often remain hidden until introspection takes place, and we can judge and re-evaluate our introjections, rather than become them.

Racism evokes a form of humiliation, both public and personal. I have worked with clients who have been entangled in shame. Shame is an intersectional oppression because it digs up the ways that we have been hurt as humans, due to oppressions and the stereotyping of what humans should be and how they should act. Humiliation therefore runs deep in cultural systems, including families and education systems.

Assimilation and humiliation work hand in hand to bring about cultural norms. These features are integrated into human behaviour that can provoke a sense of shame or humiliation. In some areas of the world public shaming is still a feature of controlling social norms. In 16th and 17th century Europe, public shaming was carried out in the form of placing a person in the stocks in a public square where they could be jeered at and be victims of scorn and humiliation from passers-by.

The public were given free rein to project their own humiliation and ideas of punishment onto the offender. Being tarred and feathered, public lynching, cutting off hands, and stoning still exist in some areas of the world. These days we have prison systems that incarcerate humans when they have been accused of wrongdoing. Within the prison walls, there are additional forms of humiliation, from peers, staff and stigmas enforced by societal norms. These stigmas are in themselves punitive and often become internalised causing the receiver to emotionally or physically harm themselves in their defence against humiliation.

Humiliation is either a feature of the mindset, a projection of someone else's shame, or their ideas of straightening up into a culturally assimilated being. This can serve to be transformative in that learning from the experience can happen, or it can mean that we are forever bound up in coping behaviours and defences to keep us from the harm that humiliation can cause. Humiliation can reinforce assimilation or throw light on attitudes and behaviours that may be disapproved of. Thus, assimilation can be forced, reinforced, inculcated, or chosen. This is where a sense of freedom is essential.

I am an assimilated British national who in the main is law abiding. I don't quite understand whether the rules I stick to are those of the ten commandments, instilled into my consciousness as a child, or whether I am naturally good, kind-hearted and caring. When I am terrified, or feeling furious and vengeful, I do not know whether I was taught this behaviour, and associated feelings or whether they arose from internalisation of my life experiences and societal rules. I do know that some of these behaviours came about because of conforming and assimilation. As an adult having experienced kindness, positive reflection, encouragement to self-love, and reciprocated care, I have an idea of what that feels like. I am no longer the abandoned, humiliated, angry child; I am conscious and aware that I have a choice to assimilate positive connections and loving, tender care. I am also aware that my conscious decisions not to assimilate can create conflict within my family and between friends and colleagues.

Recently I had a situation where I grappled with my humiliation and the confusion of attempting to assimilate. I did not understand the language in the corridors of power. I had applied for the concept of a 'black Empathic Approach' to be trademarked. I am proud of this concept and offering it for scrutinization and acceptance. I ended up challenging its refusal and making two appeals that were penultimately refused. I had not fully understood the jargonised context of the refusal. I felt humiliated. After discussions about the meaning of 'their' language of refusal, that was steeped in the law, as it was explained, I realised that there was no recourse.

Today as previously arranged I had an interesting conversation with the intellectual property office. They have refused to accept registration or as they say, 'providing a trademark' for my concept of the 'black Empathic Approach'. Of course, they were recording the conversation, and I had a friend listening in on another phone. I have a life outside of my legacy work with this approach, but I also live it.

Talking to my friends and those who appreciate what I am doing, helped me feel inspired, accepted and not alone in this task. This was a last-ditch appeal for my precious concept that is now being described in this book. It has taken a long time for practitioners to grasp what I really mean by a black Empathic Approach. That's not surprising. I am grappling with a government organisation, guarded by the law. They have no real idea where I'm coming from. I just needed an opportunity to air my concerns about the lack of openness to an ordinary person, a black woman, attempting to make a mark on the discourse of clearing up racial trauma. I understand now that trademarking a concept is a very precious step. A step in trying to prevent exploitation of my work. Something close to my heart, created from my research and transitioning into a legacy. They would not understand that I felt excluded by the jargonised messages in their refusal documents. I now fully understand that there are two keywords that I was supposed to pay elaborate attention to.

During the discussion with the officer from the Intellectual Copyright Office, I felt I was being tricked because it came to light that one thing had been said to me but really, they meant something else. I experienced a sense of elitist promise to uphold their laws of trademarking, no matter what, and that not being clear with me and twisting their descriptions meant I remained ignorant of the rules and therefore it meant that I would remain outside of their white bureaucratic gang.

These are the terms that I could not integrate into my application. The first being 'descriptive', the second being 'distinctive'. Apparently, my concept was deemed to be descriptive and therefore not distinctive as in the trademark Coca-Cola or McDonald's, where they do not mention the drink or the burger. Evidently, I put the drink and the burger into my concept, making it descriptive and therefore it was not deemed as distinctive. In doing their homework they researched the term 'black', the term 'empathic' and the term 'approach'. Splitting them up and finding dictionary definitions that created misunderstanding of my purpose. Of course, they did not get it because I expected empathy with my concern and a wish to change a discourse of denial. They paid little attention to my homework, that spanned my research, my writing, and the only Google term coined by me and linked to my name. I feel as though I have fought for this term to be trademarked, but I realise the battle is useless, because as my friend who was listening to the conversation suggested, I am not supposed to be in their gang, under the lawful jurisdiction, holding tight onto a concept that no one else is legally permitted to use. My friend also advised me that my ancestors were guiding me through this.

Eventually, I gained clarity about their version of the difference between distinctive and non-distinctive slogans. They wanted proof even though I believe the concept is distinctive; they want me to disguise it because it does not comply. They say it is devoid of any distinctive characteristics. They used dictionary definitions to pull it apart and claim conceptual ambiguity. There was no real argument. I was seeking an empathic understanding of my concept. In no way was this available and I felt as though, once again, I was up against a racist system that would not accept my proposition and my appeal for this term to be accepted, because they did not get it. Like a red flag to a bull, they tore the words 'black and empathic' to pieces.

To get appropriate help I needed to find thousands of pounds to pay to other members of their gang who would advise me to present it in a 'correct language'. Then I would have to reapply and put myself on the chopping block again. I realised that I was up against a system that wanted me to assimilate, and I did not have the language for this procedure. It felt like mental torture and elevated my rage, so I made a good decision to let go of it. I moved on to recognising that the trademark is this book, where I can share and support my reasoning for use of the concept and readers can share with me.

My friend told me that I do not need to be in that gang. I considered my reasons for wanting to join the gang in the first place and I realised that I was expecting them to accept and protect my concept from exploitation. This is intellectual discombobulation and mental slavery. My decision to let go of it and move on to recognising that trademarking it in this book makes it accessible rather than mystified and colonised. Empathy from my home girls is what I really needed. This made me feel validated and supported in my quest to bring this concept to the world. The support and acceptance from those who know my work soothed my rage.

I share this experience with readers, as an example of my discombobulation when unable to fit in with the system. I had felt helpless and incompetent and came to the realisation that unless I could fit in, the system is designed to make me feel this way and give up hope. I'm writing about it to release it from my list of things to do and to move on to the real business of a black Empathic Approach. It was naïve to expect a black Empathic Approach from a government trademarking office. Now I am aware that it was money and time wasted, and I could have been running into allowing my concept to be colonised. There has been a divine intervention whew! This term does not need to be colonised or capitalised. It is already accepted, utilised, and assigned to my precious work influencing the discourse of racism, perpetrated trauma and unattended to racism in the mental health of clients, supervisors, training and the helping professions. My learning from this experience which spans over six months, has been useful. I hope that others will learn from this too. Now on with the real work.

I have many examples of humiliation. Some of them have shown up as a mixture of racism and classism. For example, whilst teaching, the classroom door opened and a white lecturer who had clearly seen me in front of the class, called out to me 'where is the lecturer' I walked to the door and addressed her, but I wondered how the class had witnessed this incident of marginalisation and humiliation. I knew immediately she had addressed me in this way because of my skin colour, my hair, and her assumptions that all lecturers are white.

On another occasion, I was deemed to be a student by a white lecturer whilst I was using the photocopy machine in the staff room. She informed me with an authoritarian tone that 'the photocopier was for staff use only'. I was indignant and asked her whether she was a student or a lecturer. This was my way of hitting back.

At times I am a silent witness to the oppressions that come my way. Not only have I been asked if I am Jewish whilst entering the synagogue, but I have experienced a kind of imposter syndrome when the service is performed in Hebrew. I cannot speak or read Hebrew, but I can read transliterations. The first day that I was able to sing in Hebrew transliteration, having been offered this opportunity, I felt moved and connected to a part of my heritage that had long been denied me, and a hidden part of my identity. This helped me feel more confident about being the only one in a sea of white Jewish faces.

I am curious about the link between imposter syndrome, the wish to assimilate, and the fear of humiliation. Imposter syndrome is a common occurrence. It can be viewed as a feature of assimilation and humiliation. Racism, misogyny and emasculation are cogs that turn and grind in the wheel of shame, humiliation, and assimilation.

As a young child, I have memories of being removed from the bedroom, and the company of five other children and put into the empty playroom as a punishment for not staying in bed. The playroom was a large empty space. There was brown lino on the floor and the walls were cream coloured, the appearance of the room was dark and unwelcoming and the shutters across the windows were left open. I could see the bushes outside of the window waving in the dark and the lamp light shining through them, creating scary silhouettes. My mind played havoc with the silhouetted shapes and shadows on the glass that frightened me. I imagined the bogeyman waiting behind the glass to come and get me, because I had done something wrong. To this day I am afraid of being in the dark outside on my own. This lasting memory has become a source of humiliation, because often other adults cannot understand why I have this fear, until I explain what happened to me as a child.

Punishment can be seen to regulate assimilation. Assimilation patterns can become unconscious hurts or stimulate hurtful memories and shame. Humiliation can bring to the conscious mind hurtful memories of undermining, abandonment, worthlessness, chastisement and punishment. More so when a person is conscious of feeling they do not fit into an environment they have chosen to be part of.

A wish to assimilate can be entwined with experiences of 'imposter syndrome'. It is a feature of low self-esteem that may appear and come into awareness in certain situations. Repeated situations of imposter syndrome can create feelings of worthlessness. In its extreme, the subjects of this mental phenomenon may ignore validation.

The language by which we are presenting ourselves may not be the language that we really believe to be our own, in terms of presentation. Most people can claim to be assimilated into a culture within which they exist, but this does not necessarily mean they are confident in presenting themselves within that culture. Certain barriers can arise in the form of cultural misdemeanours that they had formally associated with being authentic. They may have been humiliated and misrepresented due to the prejudices of others.

Successive assimilation can cause individuals to behave as though this is an acceptable norm, nevertheless, we are still able to compete, which is a requirement of assimilation. There is stress in the corridors of power, so many individuals become compliant, and assimilation appears normal and the only option for their survival. This option is laid bare once burnout, or oppression overload becomes apparent and mental health concerns are paramount. When this happens, we become disappointed in ourselves and sometimes feel guilty about letting others down. Our assimilation is blown apart, and the downside to this breaking of the norm and respectability of assimilating can be isolation.

Internalising humiliation can lead to incongruence resulting in not feeling real, or genuine when presenting to others, or a feeling of not knowing our true selves. From this, emanates a kind of slave mentality that dwells inside the mind and persuades performances of servitude that hide the real self. Layers of assimilation can become eroded by sudden tragedies or traumas that interrupt our lives. The masks that covered our hurts and distresses become cracked, and managing the assimilation becomes difficult. A fragmented mask can expose our vulnerability and provoke a need for empathy and support. Sometimes low levels of self-care, as in putting others' needs before our own can jeopardise our own well-being.

In 2020, the world was exposed to the reality of police brutality. The US and the UK were formerly nations known as civilised, reserved and proper. The mental and emotional wear and tear of systemised racism, and the discourse of coercive assimilation within these institutions was highlighted.

After the pavement lynching of George Floyd and the upsurge of 'Black Lives Matter' arose a conglomeration of enquiries about therapy and support for training courses and groups of people working in the caring professions. Professionals were crying out for support to unravel concerns about institutional racism. Some were genuinely traumatised by the news items that suggested outrage and the critical mass of pain. There was disappointment and the need for institutional racism and statues representing oppression to be eliminated. My rage was justified by public rage, and the humiliation and isolation of being a protagonist of antiracism became lessened.

For some the evolving protests after this incident were traumatising and scary. A threat to their mental health and changes in the status quo. In psychotherapy practice and teaching, it became clear that white people expect us as black people and people of colour to lift them out of their surfacing distresses about what they have created for centuries within institutions that were built on our ancestor's backs. Professionals began to recognise their fragility and outlined the need for help. The call was out, and many responded dutifully to try and assist the perpetrator group to elevate their attitudes and save the face of a damaged system and the individuals holding it together. I called the response 'voluntary servitude'.

It was never our job to take care of the slave master or his family, but once upon a time, this role was enforced on African peoples through slavery. It's our responsibility to take care of ourselves and our own families. All things being equal. In many communities, traditionally, we show care and concern in the village. In this situation, the services of BPOC therapists and trainers were being called upon, over and above our regular duties. There was little consideration for our own self-care and well-being, given that as individuals and as communities we already carry with us into our daily lives the burdens of everyday racism and transgenerational oppression. BPOC needs to liberate ourselves should be on the backs of warriors and not by increasing voluntary servitude.

We get tired and worn down by the constant struggle to emerge from historical, intergenerational and everyday traumas instilled by racism and the cause to assimi-late, to serve others and not be fully ourselves. We're often burnt out and suffering from oppression overload. This discourse has been named 'compassion fatigue'. Levels of recovery may be influenced by economic pressures and lack of support. Pushing through this to save our lives means asking for help.

Asking for help can also feel humiliating when this is something we are not used to or may have been repeatedly refused. For most of my life I have not been used to asking for help or taking help for granted. I often look as though I'm coping when I could do with a helping hand. I call this Modus-operandi 'compulsive independ-ence'. (2) I recognise it in others, in particular black women who are accustomed to holding up the world and coping without enough support. As a form of assimilation some BPOC individuals internalised this expectation, and we just get on with it until it becomes too much for us and shows up in failing health.

The collusion of hatred and oppression of our ancestors has perpetrated ways to keep BPOC people as underlings and in servitude. This is born out once again by statistics evidencing our over representation in the mental health system and the penal system and those impacted by the outrageous Windrush scandal. The high level of BPOC who perished due to COVID-19 and lack of attention to adequate protection of health workers is tantamount to this. All this has decreased our levels of survival in the West.

The current climate of righteous indignation is a surge or catharsis from the trauma of what had been sublimated in the collective unconscious, but blatantly obvious for many sufferers and observers of this human blight. Assimilation tech-niques and defences are laid bare as we make attempts to survive the trauma of racism.

In my writing and in training I have mentioned the 'step and fetch it' and 'Mammy' archetype. Those who feel a duty to caretake individuals and groups who feel guilty about their role in maintaining the racialised status quo and oppres-sion, misrepresentation and miseducation of BPOC peoples. During the early 18th and 19th century, the image of the subservient black Mama who took care of the slave master's family was prevalent. The mammy concept is based on caretaking of white privileged behaviour by BPOC individuals, so as to protect them from the black rage of the subjects of racism.

White privileged individuals who are assimilated into racist Eurocentric sys-tems sometimes feel they are losing something by giving up their privileged posi-tions, and creating anti racist alliances with us, so that we have support to liberate ourselves, our families and our clients. They do not realise that this change also liberates them, and that systemized racism is personal, political and psychological. The recent surge to transform racist discourses is a hope that we are collectively emerging from the trauma of our past and have high expectations of rising above the intimidation, undermining and crushing collective trampolining on our peoples.

This gross situation that we have been living with in the Western world, and its effects has created mental, physical, spiritual and emotional malaise. The mentality of the privileged white has caused them to feel guilty that we have exposed this mistreatment. Now we are saying that never again will we allow them to continue their racist behaviour towards our people. Assimilation can mean that we forget that we have our own wounds to heal, and we put them aside and rush to show white people what they should do to recover from their guilt and anti-black racism.

Our personal and collective wounds from racism need to be healed so that we can look at the ways that internalised racism can cause BPOC communities to humiliate each other, betray our origins, and adopt disconnected ways of being that do not serve us. It is our job to focus on our recovery and when we feel strong enough, when the pain and tears have dissipated, when we feel loved, supported, nurtured, nourished and respected enough, then we may be ready to use our experiences and skills to inform those in the white privilege, perpetrator group on how to train themselves up and be better allies for us.

Individuals are at risk of burnout and mental ill-health if they are trying to convince themselves that this change can occur by 'Mammying'. They have made us think and sometimes act as though our brains are smaller. This is not true. They have an underdeveloped emotional capacity that has been projected onto us. Collectively they are slow in learning humaneness, and they appear to us as though inadequate and not knowing. They appear persecuted when we challenge them. This is the face of white fragility. They will come to us looking humble, wanting our pity and needing to be rescued. They are pitifully trying to make us think they do not know how to change their inadequate world of white privilege and patriarchy. We may become confused and buy into this need for care, but what are they offering us? We are intelligent people. We need to stop and consider whether we are being rewarded and compensated for our emotional, physical and spiritual labour and our achievements.

Because of our internalised racism, we become inhibited and embarrassed by their silence. It is difficult to sit with, and we jump to rescue them from their difficulties and inhibited stance of burying their heads in the sand. We want them to pull their heads out of the sand and be bold, speak out to each other, and get their act together. The pain inside us is excruciating and we want to recover from it, so we try to rescue them, and they do not learn what they need to know to help each other. We do not need to save them.

They are like unschooled children, and we need to let them be schooled, so they can learn how to live in our world peacefully and stop oppressing us. I need to speak these things so that my rage is taken seriously. When my rage is taken seriously my compassion emerges.

Drivenness and compulsive independence are components of internalised oppression, and racism. Rather than processing our rage, these components of our behaviour can force us into assimilation. BPOC were driven during slavery and indentured labour and expected to work over and above human capacity. Without rest and rejuvenation. Without this replenishment, it was difficult to see ourselves. Our gaze became distorted, and we just kept going for the survival of our people and the generations to come.

During slavery, BPOC were trained to watch each other being slaughtered, not cry out for help and we were encouraged against creating close communities that fight for each other. This is the hard face of humiliation and assimilation. This heinous lie kept us separate and subservient for centuries. We are free to end this mental slavery.

Assimilation can be culturally positive and yet it can create stereotyping, coercion and unconscious social sanctions based on humiliation. Many projections are based on assumptions about who the other person is. Understanding and accepting the ways in which assimilation can function is important to our empathic framework. Empathy is not fully honest and congruent if it is based on elements of stereotyping and assumptions. When considering a black Empathic Approach, the therapist's personal assimilation and understanding of this dynamic, coupled with the process of racialisation and experiences of racism, can function for and against their own and their clients' mental well-being. Humiliation can expose our most vulnerable and inner fears and feelings, whether it be an incident that has rolled off our backs, or whether it be something deeply shaming.

Alleyne (2022) P. reiterates that 'shame is "*relational, involving scrutiny of the self and one's identity, and can lead a person to think 'I am a bad person', or 'How could I have done that?'…. It is associated with other emotions such as humiliation, disgust, disgrace and other self-evaluating ruminations, all of which degrade and pervade all aspects of the self*" (P84). She goes on to say that *shame can be toxic and stay buried within, becoming 'part of our self-identity'. (P85) The most common precursor to this kind of shame is trauma'*. The traumatic impact of anti-black racism can be passed down generations reinforcing identity, and inferiority complexes.

Summary

The intersection between assimilation and humiliation, depends on acculturalisation, coping skills and socio-empathic responses, support and direction.

Therapists have a job to do on themselves which is to expel the negative ways they cope with daily anti-black racism. Together, we can be stronger, joyful, clear of thinking and develop a positive black gaze that reflects who we really are and gives us the opportunity to emerge from ways that are not healthy for us. We need to remember that healing from the hurts of our past as BPOC people is a priority over our teaching of the privileged group. When they do their work, we may feel more equal. We may feel less humiliated and more powerful.

Notes

1 https://australianstogether.org.au/discover-and-learn/our-history/stolen-generations.

Chapter 5

Engaging with internalised racism

UK 2023

As I start to write this chapter my heart is heavy. My first son is lying in hospital paralysed. He had a fight with the police who broke his neck. Unlike George Floyd and many others who did not survive broken necks and asphyxiation, he is still breathing. When I was notified of the disaster, knowing how tough his life had been, I questioned, had he tried to hang himself. He is now lying helpless in hospital. He can talk, he can eat if he's fed. He may never be the same again. His physical, emotional and mental needs are huge. His wounds go deep, and the system has caught him in its Eurocentric web and rendered him helpless, dehumanised and emasculated. No matter what caused the altercation, he did not deserve to be reduced to this helpless state. He is a grown man, and I am still his mother. There is a bond that keeps us as one no matter what. I feel helpless and want to preserve my own self-care, so that I can continue to be strong enough for my family and create this legacy.

I had defended my son from bullying in primary school, but the teachers didn't seem to understand what I was seeing, of their emasculation. His fighting back was just merely seen as aggression. I did not feel heard or supported by them. He was the child artist who wanted to be an architect, whose white female fourth form teacher wanted him to become an athlete. She was already stereotyping him. In his defence, I had challenged his secondary school teacher about trying to channel my child into a stereotypical stream typically assumed by a racist educational system. Things went downhill after that. Instead of embarking on A level arts, his career ended abruptly. He left school prematurely and I felt helpless as a single unsupported mother. There was no safe place for my child who had been bullied in school and by the police on his way home from school and by grown white men in public spaces.

He left home and started a career in the gym pumping iron, to make his image bigger so other men would not mess with him. His subsequent body dysmorphia and engagement with substitute fathers and the Alpha world led him to the use of ketamine and other dangerous mind-altering substances to big him up and numb his mind to the mental pain of his world.

DOI: 10.4324/9781003479994-6

He is a gentle giant and seems to have battled his way to adulthood and father-hood until now. I have always questioned how a black, female, single parent, raises her black sons to be strong and self-respecting in body, mind and spirit. Having had no father, mother or grandparents to raise me, I had no blueprint, but I've done my best. I had felt dismembered from the moment when I realised his predicament in primary school, when he was misunderstood and labelled for fighting back, when he was being bullied by other children and the white teachers. He was always aware of being singled out for his size and the colour of his skin. Being deeply connected to him, I am empathic about his predicament, and I am feeling helplessness as I call for support and justice. The empathy I feel for him is buried deep in my gut and contextually it is about surrendering to being grateful that he is still alive. I see a long struggle ahead regarding the challenge of hope for his rehabilitation.

I am aware that he is on his back in a hospital bed, in a system that has labelled him and virtually annihilated him. On my visits to the hospital, I listen to his observations of the nurses, most of whom are African, Caribbean and Asian. He can point out those who are able to care for him without bias. He cannot press the buzzer because his hands are too weak. His voice is the only tool he can use to attract help. He tells me that sometimes a black nurse will not respond when he is calling her. He challenges her disrespectful behaviour, and the reply is a stirrups (sucking through the teeth). This is a display of internalised racism and likely internalised sexism, projected at him from within a system that creates divisions between positions of power and the powerless. A black empathic approach recognises these behaviours and can identify the hurts within and between us as BPOC.

The first time I became fully conscious of being black was on a beach somewhere in Kent. A group of white traveller children, holding each other's hands formed a ring around me. I had somehow separated from the carer and the others from the children's home who were white. 'Darkie, Darkie' the chant echoed out, and rip-pled through a circle of outstretched arms surrounding me. Speechless I looked at them in bewilderment. I felt trapped and alone. The stony beach, the roar of the waves and the echo of their voices reinforced my silent incarceration. I took in that I was different, disliked and to be teased. I cannot calculate the intensity of what was being delivered to me, but I know that the rest of that outing was a blank. My carers must have been oblivious to my situation and that was that. I must have carried on as normal and pushed down inside that humiliating incident. This mode of coping with oppressions directed towards me, stayed with me for decades, until I became more self-aware and 'woke', as they say. Like many others who have suf-fered the silencing impact of racism, I have grown to recognise coping mechanisms that are more conducive to my self-care and well-being.

Internalised racism is evident where the psyche has been wounded and humili-ated by racism. This can create behaviour that may not always display evidence of this oppression. Taking for granted what we know as racism, does not mean we are equipped to demonstrate a black Empathic Approach. Therapists must know themselves and their capacity to identify where racism has been internalised. It is likely that unless clients are familiar with the language of antiracism, they may not identify their need for support with internalised racism. This is because, generally racism is experienced as covert or systemic. Internalised racism can cause shutting down and disbelief that racism has been introjected, and this can affect ways of articulating its intersecting influence on individuals.

My own experience of internalised racism feels like a permanent bruise within my heart. This manifests in my mind, being vigilant, when I'm interacting with people, whether they seem aware of the impact of racism or not. I am aware that I harbour an internal, lifelong abrasion, due to my white mother abandoning me at an early age, a wound that has never been soothed. Subsequently, the white boys in the children's home bullied and abused me. This early mistreatment amounts to a black girl, being abandoned by the white part of her family and the intersectional misogynoir and sexism experienced throughout her young life.

Tobago 2024

Yesterday I attended a forgiveness retreat that reinforced the possibility of giving up disappointment about a painful and broken past, reinforced by many relationships where I have been hurt. In addition to my regular Co counselling, the retreat has enabled me to focus on relieving myself from the pain of my internalised oppressions, and the associated patterns of mistrust, fear and rejection. I realise that I have the option to choose a new path, of letting go of those wounds and moving on to a loving, more trusting, supportive future. This realisation has connected me with sharing and gathering of experiences, and others who are making decisions about moving their lives on compassionately. I have a much stronger sense of knowing that those who hurt others operate on a downstream of their own hurt, that has nothing to do with me. My way of knowing is supported by others who believe in this knowledge and self-preservation, based on developing more joy and recognition, and that essentially those perpetrators need to heal themselves.

Hurricane Beryl is about to slay areas of the Caribbean. We have been warned of danger to our islands. Being on a red alert is a first for me. Some friends and family called me to check if I'm OK and give me supportive backup information. I felt held in their love, and so far, have arrived safely into today.

Phrases such as 'burying the head in the sand' and 'the elephant in the room', give context to situations where internalised racism creates fear, silence and numbness rather than addressing racism. I have many personal experiences of shutting down on my feelings about racism. I remember being at a conference where there were only one or two BPOC delegates in a sea of white faces. I witnessed and heard racism in the conference room. I wanted to speak up, but my heart was thumping, and the words stayed inside of me. In that moment of terror about exposing my thoughts and drawing attention to my skin colour, I was frozen. This was one of many feelings of disempowerment, that came about due to my internalised racism. The best I could do with my feelings, was to speak to someone who looked like me and who may see and hear me. By chance, they may have also noticed what had happened during the conference and possibly, been able to offer a black empathic connection. One of my lifelong coping patterns was silencing myself. Intersectionally, my numbness in the moment, was also a feature of my adolescence and early impostor syndrome, that functioned to save me from humiliation in school, when I felt I didn't know the answers.

Individuals struggling with the impact of anti-black racism often face denial and defensiveness from those around them and these responses exacerbate feelings of being abnormal in addition to the hurt of the oppression. If onlookers or perpetrators of racism are naive or rigidly protecting themselves from the challenge of this experience, they can act in ways that give the receiver cause to believe that there is something wrong with them. In addition to this the subject of these oppressions when recognising that empathy or support is not available, may develop forms of denial. Experiences of these oppressions coupled with lack of recognition or support, get layered on top of early incidents of racism. Accepting that these feelings are a normal response to an abnormal situation is key to a black Empathic Approach.

Rage, fear and guilt are feelings associated with internalised racism. A silence about these powerful feelings can create shame. Whilst being shamed and feeling ashamed individuals harbour fear about exposure to hatred and lack of appropriate coping skills that support their powerful feelings. Counteracting or challenging overt racism or supporting others experiencing racism is often seen as taboo. In turn, the powerful feelings mentioned above become internalised and can be experienced as self-stigmatisation. In other words, a person who can easily be hurt by racism. An oppression that others often do not want to address. An individual internalising to this extent is harbouring powerful feelings of recognition trauma. The isolation linked to these experiences can cause self-questioning of a person's mental health. Questions such as why am I feeling so enraged? Is there something wrong with me? Am I the only one experiencing these feelings? If an individual does not experience an appropriate empathic response to these questions, they may become disillusioned with connecting to others, resulting in isolation.

For myself, I'm always angry when witnessing experiences of racism. My self-care becomes a priority and alongside this nurturing of my soul, I am aware of when I swallow the bitter pill that leads to internalisation of the pain and humiliation. Of course, there are many factors of oppression in my life that get triggered during these experiences, and my growing self-awareness of how coping skills become dislodged when racism strikes, opens pathways to developing modes of recovery. I have a way of dipping into my toolkit of compassion. In the first instance self-compassion, self-love, nurturing and asking for help.

In therapeutic work with a group of women who have experienced the intersecting oppressions of racism, sexism, misogyny and homophobia, to name but a few, I recognised several phases of awareness, associated with the impact of racism.

Here are some examples of responses to racism and sexism and ways of using a black Empathic Approach, to identify Internalised racism.

I was taught to put my head up and get on with things.

Supporting an individual who has been instructed to ignore racism can mean unpicking some denial of their experiences and how they have managed this behaviour, whilst observing the ways that racism can come at us. The black Empathic Approach can mean learning new ways of coping rather than being numb and internalising the oppressions.

I never experienced racism, my family were very black conscious, so I had a lot of support to grow my confidence.

Individuals who are fortunate to be raised in a black conscious family can be assisted to continue growing their confidence in places where the family is not present. For example, at work and in educational situations where racism can be both covert and overt. A black Empathic Approach can reinforce confidence and assist in building strategies to cope, that break isolation and disappointment about racism in social situations.

I grew up with three brothers, so I learned very early how to handle men.

Growing up with brothers cannot be taken for granted as an approach to coping with misogynoir and other intersecting oppressions. A one-size-fits-all approach may not be a saving grace for this person. A black Empathic Approach can address this intersecting experience, whilst supporting an individual to develop an identity perspective that embraces their femaleness and self-care as a woman, prone to invisibility and undermining from the outside world.

My mother was a quiet woman, and I never saw my parents arguing.

A black Empathic Approach in this situation can be of assistance to exploring the unseen and sometimes unheard pain of a quiet woman, especially if she is a black woman who may silence herself rather than confront the oppressions. Not seeing parents argue does not mean they do not argue. Individuals may have an argument or a challenge that needs to be aired yet may be held within and become harmful and unexpressed due to feeling unsafe to share. A black Empathic Approach can assist by deepening the listening process, with someone who feels they cannot challenge, or that they have been shut down, due to internalised racism. On several occasions, I have explained to clients the meaning of 'internalised racism'. This has given language to their unspoken coping skills.

I was raised properly, and my father was very strict. everything had to be just so, or we got beaten.

The experience of being beaten as a child is controversial. Some say, "t didn't do me any harm", but then go on to beat their own children or their life partners and ignore the pain of this transgenerational form of slave mentality that comes from the past and is often justified in the present. (Slave mentality is a feature of low self-esteem, that affects how you see yourself. You always feel like you have to depend on another person. You have no self-worth, and a victim mentality. You never see yourself as a victor.) This is the difference between a person's empowerment and allowing power over themselves. As we learn more sensitivity and ways of coaching humans into non-violent, nurturing behaviours, the process of ownership and assumption that abusive behaviour is appropriate communication begins to dissipate.

A black Empathic Approach can play a part in supporting individuals to say 'No' to violent and abusive behaviour of any sort and support them to let go of rigidities that may have been instilled in them. This form of internalised racism can be counteracted by assisting the individual to develop their self-care and eliminate the harshness of physical violence.

The impact of racism and oppression on the psyche is not a new phenomenon for psychotherapy, counselling and other therapeutic practices. However, these disciplines have generally relied on traditional theories that do not always encourage an active approach to the challenge and conjoining intersections with racism. This challenge perpetuates a split that I named cultural schizophrenia (Mckenzie-Mavinga 2009. P117).

The demeaning impact of racism can be seen in limiting behaviours. For example, hiding behaviour that creates a false self, often resulting in code switching and imposter syndrome. Giving greater attention to skin lightening and hair straightening products, rather than developing pride in natural hair and ways of being, is a major enterprise perpetrated by Asian companies. These companies are selling and profiteering to black African women, instead of promoting African features as beautiful and worthy of appreciation. These products that emulate white privilege have become a distraction from the true self. This may seem a judgmental and concerning statement, but if we are to work therapeutically with internalised racism, it is important to address shadeism/colourism in all its forms, between black, African, Asian and people of colour.

It is not healthy to ignore the divisiveness and low self-esteem that perpetuates internalised racism, whether it be aesthetic or a silent enduring hurt, nibbling away at our insides and creating chronic diseases. Therapists must provide a safe space to engage with the impact of racism as an intersecting form of oppression.

Rather than ignore or glide over features of internalised racism we can lovingly and empathically engage with these behavioural concerns that so often grow with us from an early age. These wounds are retraumatised and perpetuated by Institutional and societal racism.

A client's experience of lockdown and internalised racism

One of my last clients shared the excruciating pain of living and working as a black woman in a South Asian country. During the COVID lockdown, she felt trapped within the country, within her home, and within herself. Her separation from family and cultural community was exacerbated during this period. She developed hyper-vigilance within her work as an on-screen teacher. If she was on the streets as a black woman and went out for anything other than the reasons allowed, she was at risk of being deported and therefore losing her job. She was unable to travel to visit family and friends that looked like her. She was not in a significant relationship. She was unable to get to a hairdresser.

I will call this client 'Hope'. We had been meeting online, in the therapeutic space for over a year. She worked in a school of 3000 and the parents of these children had high expectations of teachers to help their children excel. Hope felt that the clock was ticking, as she was heading towards forty and we had explored her feelings of hopelessness about finding a permanent relationship. She was born in the UK and had been sent to Jamaica as a young child and raised for a few years by her grandparents. Feelings of abandonment by her mother had created a defensive wall around her. Whilst she felt protected by the wall, it was difficult for her to feel close to her mother as an adult and imagine a new intimate relationship.

Hope was a successful teacher, the job held high esteem, but she experienced herself as the only black teacher in the school and somewhat isolated in her feelings of not being good enough (Imposter Syndrome). Her way of keeping safe meant being wary in all social situations and feeling unsure whether she was really accepted by her peers.

Her pupils loved her, and she was hard working and committed to their achievements. When COVID happened, she felt trapped in her small apartment and in the long hours of working online. She was expected to work at home for the consistency of the school curriculum, and commitment to parents. She laboured long and hard all day and too late into the evenings when she would be marking the day's work and preparing for the following day. She worked over and above the hours that were her normal everyday teaching with the children.

The rules of lockdown seemed additionally severe for this black woman, who felt under tremendous pressure to conform, because otherwise her skin colour would attract punishment. During this period, she was not sleeping well and was lacking exercise. She had been used to visiting a fitness centre, meeting friends and eating out. Her self-worth had become decreased by the experience of lockdown and her internalised racism.

There were many sessions when she expressed her fatigue and the burdensome, isolated situation that she was in. Staff meetings on screen were excruciating and made her feel inadequate, as the only black woman in her team. In some sessions, she expressed that she felt she couldn't go on. She felt emotionally and physically burnt out. She never thought she would get through this period of lockdown and having to continue homework at a more intensive level. She counted down the days when school would be out, and she could take a break from the hard labour.

As we sat looking at each other on the screen. I noticed that the extensions in her hair had become untidy after the first few weeks of staying at home. She described the untidiness of having papers scattered in her living area due to the long hours of work she was enduring, in her tiny apartment. At the end of lockdown, she explained a sense of freedom that she was feeling after having taken out her hair extensions and now wearing her hair natural. She had previously travelled to the next town to have her hair done, but with lockdown, she couldn't travel and had no opportunity to visit a hairdresser. "I would never have walked on the streets like this before our sessions", she explained. "I didn't have the confidence. I thought that my hair mattered, and I would be targeted because of my natural hair and my Brown skin". She told me, "I feel free now, and it's good to feel my scalp and natural hair". She told me of her decision not to wear extensions, because "now I feel confident and no longer afraid of what people might say or think about me as a black woman".

I sat in silence and smiled at her as she described her feeling of liberation from the confines of lockdown, and from playing herself down, because she is a black woman and because of racism. I felt a sense of pride as I listened, and my eyes filled with tears of joy and relief shared with my client. Not only did she feel liberated in her mind, but she also physically liberated herself from the mental incarceration of racism and the confinement of being in her Brown body with natural nappy hair.

I mirrored the pride that Hope expressed in her liberation and self-concept. She had changed her image because of the fear of racism and now she was living outside of the oppression and being visible without fear and with the confidence that she is ok as she is.

During our therapy sessions, we wrestled many times with her lack of confidence in me, her therapeutic mother. The battle was like that which she had described with her mother, when she recorded that whenever she wanted to connect with her mother and talk about herself, mother would take over the conversation as if it were all about her.

During our sessions, she gained the strength to say 'stop!' to her mother, whereas in the past, she would end the phone call, and this had exacerbated her isolation and feelings of hurt and rejection. Remarkably, it was her mother who eventually pointed out the 'wall' that Hope had put up between the two of them and was contributing to their communication challenges. In the sessions, we agreed to dismantle the wall brick by brick.

Her situation was like mine in that it was as though she had been compelled to raise herself independently and create a barrier that protected her from further abandonment in her early childhood, coupled with the rejection of racism and striving to succeed in the world as a single woman. It took a few years before she was able to talk about the divorce she had experienced, that had created so much pain in her adult life.

She had kept inside her shell. She was independent in her travel and had taken herself far away from the pain of family and betrayal in her marriage. She had learnt to get on with life yet there had been a burning pain inside of her. She had the resilience to get through the lockdown period and the strict rules of the community she was living in. Compliance was the way she kept herself safe. Her internalised racism conditioned her to behave and look a certain way, so she would not be picked on in a strange environment. She was successful yet she had grown a timidity inside her that had closed her heart down to the possibility of engaging in an intimate loving respectful relationship. Hope emerged from lockdown. She could see herself more clearly and I connected with a sense of freedom and the power of her new identity as a black woman, having shed some of her internalised racism.

Keval (2023) P35:

> One of the therapeutic challenges is to be able to create a space for ourselves as therapists, allowing a freedom of movement in thinking and feeling under the watchful eyes of our patients, who need to observe, emotionally 'poke and poke' us, and experience our struggle to reach them. I believe our capacity to remain curious and empathic in the face of their attempts to both use and misuse us, is ultimately what gives them a felt sense of safety, that there is enough emotional robustness in us which can enable them to bring all aspects of themselves to be understood and managed better. This in turn can mobilise their hope and courage to exercise their own freedom of movement.

There was a point at the end of our time together and with the relaxation of COVID regulations, where Hope had taken her hair extensions out. She expressed a certain kind of freedom after restricting her appearance for many years due to her fear of racism and fear of losing her status and job as a teacher, and the possibility of being ordered to leave the country. I sensed and responded to the freedom she experienced from releasing her restricted embodiment as a black woman. I was also aware that she was restricted by the levels of internalised racism, that she had adopted to feel safe in a foreign territory where she was visually conspicuous and likely to be targeted by her employers and the authorities. My knowledge about the hurt of internalised racism for BPOC individuals, supported my ability to follow Hope's challenging journey through her internalised racism and unite with her in her liberation. These were precious moments in the use of a black Empathic Approach with this client.

In my training as a psychotherapist, I was taught to encourage openness about significant stages in the life of an individual. These stages of attachment and separation were seen in the light of childhood development, such as the breast-feeding stage, walking, talking, separating from parents at the kindergarten stage, transition into school, adolescence, and adulthood.

Separation from family origins, cultural community and an 'appropriate cultural gaze' (see Chapter 7), were not really considered. I was not encouraged to work with the knowledge that my skin was brown, that I was in a minority of one in the training environment, and that I was being offered white clients to work with. Often, I became the subject of clients' curiosity in terms of my cultural origins and our skin diversity. I became acutely aware that this triggered feelings of not belonging, associated with racism. I swallowed my powerful feelings and did my best to pay attention to these clients. I knew full well that I had internalised something unpalatable. By exploring this 'recognition trauma', I realised it was internalised racism. This type of curiosity from white clients led me to question my role as someone with the capacity to assist them through their troubles and their own diversity.

This was one of the early silences I experienced in my training. I was a quiet student with plenty of internalised oppression and low self-esteem.

Supervision groups during the training, led by a white supervisor dismissed and silenced my attempts to address this dynamic. Having experienced abandonment as a young child. I silenced myself as a defence against the corridors of white privilege where I experienced what is now seen as imposter syndrome, because I did not feel I belonged in an institution that did not reach out to me and help me feel welcome and heard. At that time, I was dissuaded from viewing my diversity as important in my learning as a therapist. My internalised oppressions grew into a critical mass, that caused me to disengage with the learning process of sharing my story with peers and the facilitators. I had repeated this process many times throughout my education.

Sometimes I was challenged by individuals who assumed that I was bringing in an issue that seemed challenging, and impossible to address and did not belong to their learning process. This concern was difficult for students of all backgrounds. For many, there had been no blueprint for addressing the pain and trauma of racism.

There was a gay white man in my process group, and we formed an alliance based on empathy about being the only one in the village. The alliance could only go as far as sharing feelings of our respective oppressions, isolation and not being recognised in the group. In the wider course group, I was alone in a sea of whiteness without an obvious ally. Silence did nothing for my lack of trust in being held by the group and its facilitator.

On becoming a lecturer and observing this scenario with other students of colour, I became wiser and wanted to support this area of their learning. I refer to this scenario as being psychologically gagged. Somehow my empathic responses became elevated and alongside this, I grew more compassionate. I am curious about how silence as a patterned form of internalised racism gets transferred into therapeutic process and engagement. It is essential to unpick the places in a therapeutic dialogue where silence invoked by white privilege and the presence of racialised experiences can traumatise both the giver and receiver of support.

A question regarding this type of scenario, posed by a white counselling trainee during my early research is presented below:

> How do we avoid stepping into a socially conditioned posture of white racism, overtly or covertly, in the therapeutic dyad, and avoid the socio-political implications of race, by focusing solely on psychological process?
>
> (Mckenzie-Mavinga (2009) P35)

There is no blueprint for undoing socially conditioned white racism. This trainee is grappling with her internalised racism, that is socially conditioned. I cannot give her an answer to this question, because she is bound up in being told what to do, rather than exploring her levels of white privilege and how she might consider working with the impact of racism on a client. It appears she may be separating the implications of racism from psychological processes, when it is likely to be deeply embedded. Racism is personal, political and psychological; therefore, therapists need the flexibility to approach the hurt of this oppression holistically and, therefore, remain an essential part of the dynamic between therapist and client.

The inevitability of trauma as a feature of internalised racism can be linked to bad feelings that go with skin colour classification. This would have seeped into the mental system from an early age and been repeated in different forms throughout life, therefore transferred into the counsellor's psyche. Individuals pondering on this question would have created coping systems, some of which would have masked their true feelings about the situation, as well as the individuals, and institutions perpetuating anti-black racism. The example of client 'Hope' presented earlier, demonstrates how staying with the client's internal and external experiences of racism by offering a black Empathic Approach, helped the client through her internalised racism and a troubled family dynamic to experiencing her authentic self as a black woman.

At the age of thirteen, a girl who shared the dormitory of five, in the children's home, where I lived, called me a 'black monkey'. That one hit home like a furnace in my belly. I withdrew the belt I was wearing around my pretty pink skirt and with my right arm slung it backwards, with a force. The belt lashed down on Jenna's back. I don't know how many strokes were administered, but I knew that I was unleashing something that lay deep inside me. Revenge was sweet and it never happened again. More's the pity, there were no staff present to assist myself or the protagonist through this traumatic event. We were left to our own devices. Two children of Jewish descent, one white and one black, with no education on racism or anti-Semitism. This situation dissolved and I was never subject to such a brutal attack again. One wonders how children can be educated and allowed to rage about these oppressions, without damaging themselves or the oppressors.

Looking back on this event. I realise that my action, whilst releasing immediate tension and hurt, was not witnessed by any adults, who perhaps, with awareness could have comforted both of us and educated us as to how we could cope with the internalised feelings that caused such violence between us. No one came to investigate the scuffle, and neither she nor I gained reprimand nor comfort since that day. That was that. She never insulted my skin colour again, and I carried a vengeance and sadness that a part of me was hated by others, and that adults were oblivious to the tirade of oppression that I experienced as a black parentless female child, in a care home. These are the seeds of the internalised racism layered within me.

When taking a black Empathic Approach, I encouraged students to reflect on their early engagement with racist experiences and build the courage to use this as a pathway to engage with clients' experiences of racism. In other words, if you did not have an opportunity to use support to move through the pain of racism, do it now, so that you have a better grasp of how you can encourage clients to track these experiences and reform the impact that repressing the pain has had on their lives. This is the essence of working with internalised racism.

Internalised racism can co-create an intersectional backup with other oppressions. In my own identity development, I am fully aware that being raised Christian when I am Jewish and being raised in a Eurocentric environment is a default in how I have perceived myself and how others perceive me. I've had experiences of attending a Shule on a high holiday and being asked, 'are you Jewish?' I am fully aware this questioning has happened because of my brown skin. I was fully aware that my white Jewish peers were not being asked this question. I have enough internalised racism and internalised antisemitism in me to notice the powerful feelings this evokes. Reflecting on my personal therapy whilst in training, I noticed that I was seen as a black woman, while my Jewishness remained hidden. I prioritised the painful experiences of racism, sexism and misogyny that emerged in my personal development process. My Jewishness was not attended to, until several years later. As a result, these elements of my identity remain hidden and I filter them, depending on levels of safety in groups that I engage with. This is another dimension of working with intersectionality.

Breathing new life into my existence as an elder is a golden opportunity. I refuse to accommodate stereotypical ideas about the ageing process and other parts of my identity. I pay great attention to my physical and emotional needs. I am discovering the true meaning of rest and listening to my body, because I only have one. I have a greater awareness of spiritual clues that guide me, and I have a greater dependency on divine Reiki energy. I am grateful that I have time to wake up at sunrise and enjoy birdsong in a warm place. I show gratitude and ask for guidance from my guardian angels and the almighty.

Tobago 2023

This morning, I noticed there was new life. The hen nesting outside my door revealed four chicks that she had been keeping safe under her wings. I am observing a mother child relationship that I have no memory of myself. She has been sitting alone on the eggs, laid against the garden wall, behind an Agave plant, carefully protected from predators. Another single parent, I think. She has been keeping the eggs warm for approximately three weeks. I do not check the calendar, but I have a sensitivity about when her chicks were likely to be born.

I am not a pet lover, but I'm becoming more aware of my growing sensitivity to plants, animals and insects and the role that other beings contribute to the environment. I guess it's because I have a greater sense of sustaining life, saving the environment and my own personal development being influenced by the naturalness of animal family life. I spend a good deal of time watching survival programmes and noticing the natural empathy between animals in the wild. Giraffes and elephants in the wild, group and support mothers when giving birth, as though in a collective maternal process. I notice how the herd protects and safely guides the young. I am more aware of village life and community in my Tobago home, because individuals are aware of my movements, as though watching over me. These experiences were not present in my former life, but somehow, I have developed an inner resource as a parent and therapist, and I continue to work through my rage. A black Empathic Approach was seeded from these experiences.

A black Empathic Approach incorporates an understanding of internalised racism from an early age to adulthood. The elements that layer within internalised racism can be clearly seen in levels of recognition of trauma and lack of attention to the intersecting hurts of racism. This amounts to an inappropriate gaze and lack of appropriate attention to identity development and what this means for both subjects and perpetrators of anti-black racism. Whilst I am not an expert on the white gaze, I believe that competence in offering a process that engages with 'recognition trauma' for both perpetrators and subjects of racism will be useful in tackling the damage and trauma that racism can cause. This includes the damaging nature of internalised racism for both groups. Not an easy task I might say as many humans are saturated in elements of racism. These elements show up in a variety of different ways that can distort ideas of personal power between people, and power over peoples.

It is important not to forget that anger features in internalised racism. If there is no safety and no understanding of how our anger manifests, why we are angry, and what we do with our anger, we may not be clear about how to self-care for this element of humanness and often justified emotion. Righteous indignation and the ability to challenge injustice is a key human right. A black Empathic Approach would incorporate ways to facilitate anger about racism, rather than allow it to fester in the human mind and body. Not attending to this credible emotion could amount to collusion.

Lorde, (1977) cited in UCONN (2024) P6 'The response to racism is anger'

My response to racism is anger. I have lived with that anger, ignoring it, feeding upon it, learning to use it before it laid my visions to waste, for most of my life. Once I did it in silence, afraid of the weight. My fear of anger taught me nothing. Your fear of that anger will teach you nothing, also.

((2007) P124)

Lorde's acknowledgement of anger suggests that we can be burdened by our anger, if we are silenced or alone in it. I suggest that robustness to offer facilitation of anger, as a component of the black Empathic Approach, means looking at ways we process our own anger about racism. My continuous journey on this route features in ways that I am learning about my ability to offer compassion. I cannot foresee the end of the road, as I am a work in progress.

Aspects of power over different groups, communities, and land is an age-old practice carried for generations, and influenced by religious affiliation, and land colonisiation. Recent examples of this are the needless violence, killings, ethnic cleansing, warring and annihilation of land and human rights shown up in the Russian Invasion of Ukraine (2022) and the Israel-Palestine crisis (2023). In the meantime, indigenous peoples on African and Asian continents continue to have their land pillaged, and communities rendered starving and homeless. Previous wars have left communities and individuals injured, homeless, starved, traumatised, and afraid. Having worked with refugees and asylum seekers, I feel helpless about these violent systems that injure humans physically and mentally. They demonstrate power and powerlessness, dehumanisation and destruction carried out on innocents, under the supervision of men. These actions result in a lack of compassion, empathy and tenderness. Where compassion does not live, there is little room to develop a black Empathic Approach. On the other hand, I am hopeful that the numbness and trauma of internalised experiences of racism can be healed.

Summary

Powerful feelings connected to racism can become internalised and lay dormant until safety to unravel them becomes apparent. With an acceptance and understanding of internalised racism, a black Empathic Approach can provide this safety. When unravelling these feelings, a secondary layer of feelings such as shame, isolation and anger can emerge. Once a BPOC client has been supported to notice these feelings, it may be possible to celebrate their emergence from silence and to build greater confidence in their identity. In the case of a white client emerging from their privileged position and noticing the power of their colonial heritage. Guilt, anger and shame may manifest, and once this process is worked through, it may be possible for greater self-confidence to articulate knowledge of anti-black racism, and challenge racism.

Chapter 6

Being white hurts

2024 begins with a mixture of hope and hopelessness. My injured son is still lying in hospital. Movement in his limbs are limited but there are signs of his body coming back to life. He waits for the go ahead to be transferred to Stoke Mandeville Hospital, where he may be supported in the next stage of his rehabilitation. He has been quietly co-operative with the medical team, but it has not been easy. I can tell by our conversations that his feelings are un-numbing, and he wants justice for the trauma, racism and emasculation that he has experienced.

I've contacted the Cherry Groce foundation, and I'm awaiting further discussion with them in support of challenging the injuries caused by the police. I am reading the book written by Lee Lawrence, Cherry Groce's son, who witnessed the shooting of his African Caribbean mother, by a white policeman. The injury paralysed her. Lawrence (2020) 'The Louder I will sing'. Although I am trying to manage my own health issues, I am more determined than ever to write this part of my story and continue living a black Empathic Approach.

I am not well versed in white pain associated with anti-black racism. The number of white friends in my life are limited. I cannot say they are lifetime friends because our contact has been sparse. In some ways I have kept them at arm's length, due to my lack of trust and fear of their inherent racism. I am beginning to allow myself to trust more, and I count the times I feel grateful for their acknowledgment and support. Close friendships in this area are slowly progressing. I believe it's because we have had to overcome the challenges of their racism, and lack of empathy about how racism traumatises us as BPOC individuals. I do not wish to be petted or tokenized; However, I am constantly aware of how easily conflict can arise, if I am brutally honest about my need for perpetrators to become more aware and act with empathy and compassion for our communities. There is no blueprint for this area of progress, because anti-black racism also prevents insightful ways to assist white people through this dilemma.

I have researched ways to articulate, explore and create alternatives to mutually support, process and attend to powerful feelings that anti-black racism evokes. Creating safe spaces to put attention on 'recognition trauma' became a key component of the 'black Empathic Approach'. It is a tool that can bring about transformation of attitude and behaviour regarding the impact of racism. There is no

DOI: 10.4324/9781003479994-7

blueprint for this training, because it requires leaders in the field to see the need for change in attitude from the top down. A sculptor friend once said to me, that to rebuild something you must first break it down. Builders' artists and creators know the importance of taking courage to break something down and rebuild it with tougher, more appropriate and durable materials. This is the context that I am considering.

Having worked with statutory and voluntary organisations on change, with regards to institutional racism, it has become clear where the power for change lies. Investment to break down the impact of white privilege must be seen as a priority in systemic change. This is fundamental to class systems that maintain poverty, ignorance and inadequate pathways to environmental and human involvement in the manifestation of cultural confidence.

In therapy training, we are taught about reflecting, paraphrasing, mirroring and providing a gaze that supports others to see themselves. We are taught to create a knowing that reflects self-understanding and new ways of being, that build congruence, self-love, positive life relationships, and confidence. Whether white therapists offering congruence and mirroring, while harbouring hurt systemically projected onto BPOC peoples can genuinely offer an appropriate mirroring process, is questionable.

Teaching that solely reflects monocultural Eurocentric perspectives, and facilitators, who did not grow with awareness of the limitations of their training have been disenfranchised, via academic and sociocultural learning. These conditions have coexisted alongside white privilege and internalised racism. They undermined emergence from the colonial, cultural and racialised preconditions of Slavery and colonialism.

Patel (2023) P246. Notes that, 'On having worked with many organisations, some all-white teams',

> the fallacy of offering training and services based on the Western concept of self, and specifically a white, middle class, heteronormative identity, leading to professionals struggling to work with issues of race, culture and discrimination, has meant they are unprepared to work with these issues in the consulting room as they were not addressed in their training.

Consequentially the deeper explorations of how culture, race and racism have fundamentally affected the formation of the psyche, and identity at an unconscious level, are often missed. 'They did not allow space to explore and elevate individuals and their respective groups to reckon with the damage caused by these discourses, and therefore willingness to work through the trauma imposed was unlikely to be measured or supported'. This caused silence within training and therapy provision. I cannot underestimate the need for willingness to emerge from this silence as fundamental to a black Empathic Approach.

Every step of the way I am conscious of the need to create compassionate responses, whilst at the same time nurture a turning point for perpetrators of anti-black racism. Although I am aware that it is not the job of BPOC individuals to teach perpetrators, this massive task must be approached with care and consideration for traumatisation on both sides. In coming through the intensity of my rage about racism, I am seeing more clearly where a black Empathic Approach can also be utilised by white individuals who are willing to make this shift. Breaking the silence of anti-black racism is the first and most important element of growing through this dilemma.

Being white or white identified, can hurt differently for a person of colour, who can be hurt by an attack aimed at them because they are other than white. Just as the pain and prejudices associated with being male can hurt differently to those of being female.

There are similarities and differences between the pain experienced by a white person, a brown skinned person and a person whose heritage is associated with being black African or Asian and a person of colour. These very identifications based on skin colour are divisive categories, yet within those groups, they can be positive and supportive, if collusion or hierarchical skin tones, hair texture and other human features do not become blockages to connection.

White privilege plays an essential role in the divisive and painful nature of anti-black racism. I do not wish to homogenise or stereotype, but this is my way of describing what I know of white people hurting, as a feature of racism. From my position as a person of colour and black woman, I find this painful to witness, and sometimes difficult to empathise with. In thinking out loud about this, I am concerned about my own lack of training for providing this service to perpetrators of anti-black racism. It is my growing compassion that leads me to understand the need to address this area and incorporate it into a black Empathic Approach.

Andrews, K. (2023) describes a white Psychosis that invades social systems like a germ. He offers insight into the ways that whitening can swarm systematic educational provision, and saturate teaching in patronising and class driven ways. He is brutally honest about the lethargy and deliberate undermining of confidence in black studies, and the lack of meaningful ways to empower young people's identities. He pulls no punches in his description and understanding, drawn from empirical observations and his family experience.

Using his knowledge of consistent hidden data, and social policies that prevent antiracist progress and access to the best education, jobs and housing for black peoples, he proposes that the twisting of privilege to the benefit of white peoples perpetuates racism in ways that suggest black people are responsible for their lack of progress, rather than racism. What more can be said about the cultural psychosis that permeates these projections and reinforces anti-black racism.

In my Doctoral studies, white students displayed fear and guilt. Fear of being labelled racist and guilt at recognising their historical role in the perpetrator group.

In book one Mckenzie-Mavinga (2009) I named this 'cultural schizophrenia'. It is a deep historical and cultural wound that cultivates and reinforces anti-black racism.

I have never heard a white person admit to being hurt because of their skin colour. I have heard white people associated with black people, by family or friendship, expressing vicarious pain associated with those close to them. I too have been hurt by friends and family who do not look like me. Starting with my mother, a white Ashkenazi Jew, who had married a black man and produced children of colour. She was clearly hurt by the prejudice of her white family. Her intersecting oppressions of being part of a blended immigrant family who fled Nazi Europe would have been triggered.

I remember a rare occasion while visiting my mother as an adolescent. We were on a bus standing on the lower deck. My mother was in front and three small siblings behind her. Someone on the bus was pushing past us. My mother turned and exclaimed. 'Do not touch them, they are mine'. It became clear to me that in the public eye, we were disassociated from her, as a white woman unless she claimed us.

White people are undoubtedly associated with the perpetration of slavery and colonialism. These past misdemeanours are installed in their heritage and early intergenerational and transgenerational life. Similarly, black African heritage people are associated with victims and survivors of Western slavery in Africa. The denial of this historical legacy can add to hurt in the present time.

The deep hurt and numbness of white people's pain as witnesses to physical, mental and spiritual crimes against black and brown people created their own form of internalised racism. I would deem this form of white internalised racism as collective self-harm, often unconsciously projected on those who do not look like them. My mother claimed me and this unique experience of a white adult protecting my back, has not happened since.

Throughout history, notorious personal and systemic overt and covert methods of white people instilling their bad feelings about skin colour into their descendants, peers and colleagues have been noted. These unhealed hurts, projected at BPOC communities, have perpetuated anti-black racism throughout both black and white communities. When challenged about these attitudes, white people often respond defensively and without empathy. These situations challenge their ability to offer a black Empathic Approach. They question whether racism exists. They argue the validity of experiences of anti-black racism when shared. They sink into white fragility and want attention on their own hurts.

This positioning of their own need for attention and their misunderstandings about the pain of racism, often get in the way of noticing their humanness, and the humanness of the subjects of white privilege and racism. White privilege has promoted perspectives of black people that conjure ideas that we do not have feelings valid on a 'normal spectrum' of self-expression. This perspective means that our feelings and experiences do not consistently get seen or heard in a context of white disenfranchisement and unexpressed harmful elements that anti-black racism perpetuates.

Defensiveness about this perspective has caused a further chaotic road map of the experiences of BPOC people. Assumptions that form the basis of white privilege could be considered a mental health issue, in similar ways that they mess with the mental health of BPOC people. White fragility, a phenomenon now discussed more openly, has become a phase of personal development that white individuals encounter when their privilege is confronted. This is why it is necessary to unpick colonial heritage white responses to the challenge of racism. Obviously, this cannot happen unless willingness to go there and sit with the pain and privilege of having white skin occurs. This is an essential part of therapy training for white therapists.

Layers of this privilege are a key element when exploring the perpetration of institutional and personal experiences of racism. These layers are also installed into the mental DNA of mixed racial heritage and light skinned individuals.

Becoming aware of that privileged part of me as a light skinned black woman has given me insight into my positioning as an agent of oppression, and the ways that I can support, collude with, or further oppress darker skinned people. I am also aware of how perpetrators of anti-black racism expect me to collude. This challenging and complex internal engagement, that can remain unconscious, if not attended to during therapy training and personal development, can add to a mind-blowing mental disability in therapeutic work.

We can deduce that white privilege therefore cannot be solely attributed to white people. It is a system co-opted into training and educational approaches. This perspective also becomes internalised by BPOC individuals. It cannot compare with black privilege, which has its own system of internalised racism. White privilege is a system of coercion, by gradation of skin tone, that has reigned for centuries, positioned on inclusion and exclusion. Privilege is not just about economic status and power positions. It can be viewed as an internal attitude, sometimes deemed to be an 'unconscious bias'. The use of this term does not support a black Empathic Approach unless racism is explicitly addressed as both unconscious and conscious features in the relational process.

Someone who has assumed privilege can appear arrogant or collusive about oppression towards another person appearing or deemed to have a lower status. The racism that white people internalise gets projected as a privilege. Defences that accumulate from this internalisation, equivalent to deep unresolved hurt, are projected onto those with darker skin, who are assumed to be underprivileged.

In Chapter 1 my former supervisee, Anne explains the hurt within, that she had come to recognise as compounded by her racism.

She explains how white fragility, as part of that system, remains a defence against responsibility and change. A transformation from acknowledgement of systemic racism to courageous engagement with other ways of illuminating the damage that racism can do to the psyche, is necessary for change. Although slow in coming, the need for this process in therapeutic engagement and supportive contexts remains ongoing.

Cooper (2019. P203) suggests that 'white rage is deeply connected to a fear of losing privilege and status in a browning American empire. When your entire worldview is predicated by being on top, sinking from the top even a little bit can feel like an annihilation'.

Empathy is 'communication with fresh and unfrightened eyes, viewing the other person's world and experience, without judgement or prejudice'. Rogers (1959) in Clark (2023. P11) on being empathic, 'to perceive the internal frame of reference of another with accuracy and with the emotional components and meanings which pertain thereto as if one were the person, but without ever losing the "as if" condition' (PP210–211). I question whether this take on being empathic is realistic for those who have not directly experienced anti-black racism, and remain unconscious of their own internalised racism, and racist projections. I suggest that deep introspection, honesty and repair work is needed for the perpetrator group to achieve a black Empathic Approach that can be offered to others.

Of course, empathy is contextual depending on the situation and cultural reference points of those offering their reflective understanding. For empathy to be effective, the response needs to have a meaningful and emotional context. Humans are born sensitive to their surroundings. We react to loud noises; we react to gentle sounds. We react to physical touch and emotional connections, whether they be harsh or gentle. These are conditioned by cultural norms and intergenerational coercion. We grow to notice our conditioning and how that may affect our inner and outer responses to other humans and animals. Our conditioning and our responses regulate our fight or flight mechanisms, so our trauma levels may control how much we can express the empathy factor of our trust levels and expressions of deep connections to others. If therapists are not aware and emerging from their fears, they may remain unconscious of their empathy levels and ability to express empathy in different situations.

I have witnessed trainee counsellors tentatively paraphrasing the hurt of racism rather than leaning into this experience as real and worthy of expression and elucidation. Whilst experiences of other oppressions can be directly related to and empathised with, this question of how to respond to what we know is being expressed as anti-black racism has been lingering for decades. There is no hierarchy of oppressions, but often, due to rage, fear, and internalised racism, these experiences of intersecting oppressions are not always managed well. Overcoming fear of engaging with the powerful feelings that anti-black racism evokes ('Recognition trauma' Mckenzie-Mavinga 2009) is essential to a black Empathic Approach.

I question, how am I supposed to trust the use of empathy as a Eurocentric concept? If you have empathy, how could you ignore the historical impact of colonialism? If your ancestors enslaved an eight-year-old child, could it be true that intergenerationally white people do not have an appropriate level of empathy for offering sincere levels of connection with individuals impacted by anti-black racism? Therefore, becoming robust in the delivery of a black Empathic Approach would clearly have different meanings for white individuals.

Eddoe Lodge (2018) clearly exposed the difficulties of trusting white people to listen, accept and be supportive of how BPOC are gaslit and oppressed by racism. Her book (2018) titled: *Why I'm No Longer Talking to White People About Race*, attracted wide readership and attention, because she was courageous in making personal statements about the damaging effects of white privilege. It is common for BPOC Individuals to feel hopeless about telling their stories to white individuals. In the underbelly of anti-black racism, lies the unprocessed hurt that many white people do not acknowledge. Their hurt about their own skin colour and features, becomes apparent when they lie unprotected in the sunshine. When they go to tan their skin, as a means of beauty treatment. When they plump up their lips and backsides, with Botox and fantasise about having African features, in order to look more attractive. Their white privilege is dramatised by envious thoughts and the measuring of our skin shades and features against their own.

Most Western therapists and their supervisors have experienced training, built on white privilege and Eurocentric philosophic ideals. This has been damaging to the ways that therapists present themselves. How does this then compute the experience and training of black therapists? In many cases, internalised racism would have been further suppressed, undermining the care and support of their well-being. My own experience in training demonstrated that I needed to boost my education by absorbing black literature and involvement in events that nourished my self-esteem as a woman of colour. These methods backed up my personal development.

The surge of attention to 'Black Lives Matter', demonstrating we have had enough of being ignored and subservient to colonialism, meant that theoretical contexts of sociology and psychology needed to be decolonised and transformative perspectives about BPOC reinforced, with knowledge of cultural context and ways of elevating from racism.

Using the concept of a black Empathic Approach, means fully embracing a sense of healing for the black psyche hurt by racism. This also means attending to the white psyche damaged by inherent association with slavery and colonisation. Attention to the fear, sometimes even terror of changing this modus operandi and forming a different attitude towards healing the hurt of racism can then become a priority.

Here I am demonstrating where I have come to a place in my own professional and personal development that helped me to recognise the need for expansion of a generic empathic approach. I believe that if this understanding of what is needed, when attending to anti-black racism in the therapeutic sense is not catered to, there remains an ethical gap in the relational process. This is an invitation for deliberate change and application of an appropriate therapeutic method. This method requires a change in attitude and thinking and a will to apply new ways to address the traumatic impact of racism.

We don't know if empathy is innate, yet it is possible to be sensitive and intuitive to how others feel and experience their personal journeys. Empathy is something we can develop and choose to convey or not, rather than take for granted. It is important to question how essential empathy is in therapeutic contexts and be aware of how we use it. This product of human connection can be influenced by cultural conditioning. If young children experience stoicism from parents and conditioning that suggests feelings are not to be expressed, they can grow with a demeanour of not showing their feelings. This can be seen in mythology about the 'boys don't cry' approach and may bring about powerful exposure of feelings and expression, of anger and grief.

On another level, the history of racism shows that white people were taught not to show their feelings with regards to the harm done to black people. Images of white families engaging in festivities whilst observing lynchings are evidence of this. In the pavement lynching of George Floyd, white police officers observed without attempts to rescue or challenge the brutality of the scene. In the US and in the UK, there have been few charges against police officers who have participated in maiming or killing black people in the line of duty. I tried to locate data supporting evidence of UK police brutality, but I found the term 'misconduct' has been used to fog statistics on these allegations and the outcomes.

I'm determined to revisit the question of how, as BPOC, can we carry out a black Empathic Approach and come out unscathed. I guess the answer is that this may not be possible because we are human. We hurt, we project, we introject and many of us did not learn how to manage the racism experienced in our lives. We just coped.

Anne, whose acknowledgement of her deep-seated racism in Chapter 1, is fully aware of the need to work on this 'lifelong process'. She is aware of the discomfort this causes her; therefore, she will be aware of the discomfort for her clients when addressing their experience of anti-black racism. Her words portray acceptance of the hurt and intersecting oppressions deep within herself, and the necessity of opening this wider perspective. It seemed that an 'appropriate gaze' that was not sugar-coated or fuelled with guilt and shame encouraged her to delve into these places and get on with her own emergence from the pain of racism. This modelled a way of challenging and supporting her clients to explore their whiteness.

Ryde (2009): in her lecture on 'White Identity' in Psychotherapy: asks the question, 'Can dialogic, intersubjective, psychotherapy help white people work more effectively in a racialized context?' She encourages white therapists to become more aware of their whiteness. She refers to being white in a racial context, something she says she 'rarely considers'. She discusses her privilege and lack of awareness. Within the privilege is the assumption of 'white as normal'. She noticed that her white peers viewed this as coming from her experience as a white liberal. I understand this as external resistance to her research quest as opposed to support of her cause. She says that 'whiteness is not just about culture'. 'Whiteness confronted me as a stark reality'. She recalls her white working-class background as 'feeling less than', whilst being in the perpetrator position.

Ryde focuses on feelings of guilt about hurting others, and then proceeds to discuss shame. Shame is a prominent feature in revelations of racism by white people. If we are to build a black Empathic Approach that supports white people, can we consider the shame and guilt that they often express when revealing their racism? How does this sit with the black therapists internalised racism? What gets evoked and restimulated? I ask myself. Can I empathise with this aspect of recognition of trauma? Can I put my own projections and discomfort aside and remain completely present for this person? How much white guilt and shame can I endure while offering a service that may assist introspection and transform white perspectives?

She analyses her perspectives from the experience of being white, whereas my perspectives come from having brown skin, being raised as an orphan and becoming hypervigilant about not belonging. I value these experiences that formulate my perspective on a black Empathic Approach. I can get up, brush myself off and start again each day. This position has been foremost in gaining confidence, that tells me I am on track with my work and the creation of this text about a black Empathic Approach.

Ryde does not directly refer to white people hurting from the pain of white racism. Although she suggests a holistic approach that includes emotional context, she offers pointers using research and theoretical perspectives that support clearer thinking about white privilege. When Ryde alludes to white privilege that underpins racism and all its nuances, she is opening awareness of systemic racism and personal racism. This does not directly address the traumatic impact of racism. She discusses guilt and shame, and they are components of recognition trauma. Leaning into these emotions from a white perspective is fundamental to a black Empathic Approach. They are not just emotions that can be named generically as it is important to offer selective process, in the context of anti-black racism and heal its deep, festering wounds from a perpetrator's perspective.

The occurrence of offering process to the hurt that white people experience is a dynamic part of a black Empathic Approach. Shying away from a process of intellectualising can amount to collusion. Therefore, it is important to remember that a black Empathic Approach is active in addressing the hurt of racism both for perpetrators and subjects. It is an active proposition to work through the pain and trauma of racism harboured and assembled throughout life.

Interview with Anne. (Some of these questions may be useful in training contexts with white therapists)

I: *When did you first become aware of your skin colour as a white woman?*
A: I've always known I was white because I've always had friends of other races. However, I don't think I was aware of everything that came with being white regarding privilege, being a part of the problem and the impact of racism, until I was in my early 20s. One of my earliest memories is when I was four, having a kid in my preschool class who was Mexican. I inherently knew that, because he was brown, he would feel different to everyone else. I wanted to befriend him because I didn't want him to feel alone.

Between the ages of five and seventeen, my school was about 60% white and 40% black. It wasn't until I was in my late 20s, when I read something to the effect of, we view white as the norm and everything else is other, that I really started to understand. (This was either your book or 'Why I'm No Longer Talking to White People About Racism') I had grown up with the concept of difference; we were taught very well about slavery when I was age 6–8, but I couldn't have equated it to my black friend being treated differently now, because of slavery, 300 years ago. I was born in Ohio and then at 18 moved to Chicago.

I: *When did you first notice your whiteness and become aware of white racism? a) How did this feel?*

A: One of my neighbours, we cannot confirm this, but we are pretty sure, he was a member of the KKK. It was the first time I had ever heard a white person use some of the words that I had always heard that white people use. I was around 8-10, I had never heard them myself. It felt uncomfortable. He would say some disgusting things. I remember at the time being completely shocked and telling my mom. She was completely shocked and had a talk with me about how we wanted to handle it if we heard people speaking like that. It was quite scary to hear and brought home the danger that racism created.

I: *Would you say that you have felt hurt by white racism?*

A: I reflected a lot about this question and the answer kind of came to me in a moment when I was in Uganda, and I was sitting in traffic. A lot of people told me that in the capital, keep your doors locked. I was thinking, why are white people scared of everything? I was thinking about dancing and movement that I've seen around the world. A traditional dance in Africa or Latin America or Asia versus Europe. The way we clothe ourselves and the way we treat our bodies, the values we have around bodies and people in general; I was thinking that we, as a race, are afraid of everything and that's what all this boils down to. Not all of it, but a lot of it. I think we are afraid of the difference of "the other". I got really sad for myself, because I was thinking how much fear have, I internalised? I feel sad even saying it, because of the magnitude of that. It's still a new thought, like from last week. That is something to be mourned.

I: *Where would you say that fear, or that terror, if you like, has come from for white people?*

A: We lost touch with ourselves and in losing touch with our own intuition, feelings and understanding, everything became scary. We needed to create something more concrete. We needed to create a morality that was right or wrong, good or bad. We created a binary in ourselves and in creating that binary we've had to make ourselves the good ones, otherwise we would have to face our own discomfort. The fear cycle is self-perpetuating, but I think what we're most afraid of now is facing discomfort from generations of racism. The idea of framing racism as a diagnosable disorder.

I: *In the book, 'The Psychosis of Whiteness', (2023) Khinde Andrews, breaks it down as a sort of germ, like the disease. If it's a germ or a virus, then it incubates, and gets passed on. That's what has happened. In his own way, he is looking at it. Each part of how racism operates as a kind of psychotic episode for the white race. You can't really dispute it because he takes colonialism as the underbelly of all racism and breaks it down and gives facts, even to show that this is not normal and that it has been created.*

A.   Yes that's a form of madness, I do think about it like that. I'm going to love that book. I think it's an important context for understanding what has happened here and also understanding why BPOC get labelled 'psychotic' more than white people, because we take white as sane or normal.

I: *in what ways did you experience the hurt? Physical? Emotional? Were you able to talk about it with anyone?*

A: When I think about the physical aspect of this pain, it's a hollow, sinking feeling that hits like a hard punch to my chest. It comes with guilt, shame, and a warm flush to my face as well as a desire to hide. To resist this, feels like having to crack myself open and make myself vulnerable. I also know that that eases somewhat with practice, but will probably never fully go away, so it's a discomfort I must embrace and learn to recognize. I didn't have the words for that in the past, so I didn't have any way to speak to someone, but I do now. I have other white friends doing this work and it's so helpful to be able to bounce feelings and thoughts off them.

I: When was the first time that you openly supported a black or brown person experiencing racism? a) when did you first challenge racism? b) What was it like?

A: I took a road trip with a black friend to Canada. We got stopped at the border and questioned. They pulled us both out of the car to inspect it. They thought we were carrying drugs; they had very specifically questioned us. They separated us for more questioning. At this moment I can't imagine what he was feeling then, but I remember saying to the border guard, you've pulled us over because he's black. You're searching our car for drugs because he's black. They said, "It doesn't matter why we're searching your car." I said, "It does matter why you are searching our car and I need you to bring my friend back to the room." They kept us separate. I did not have the understanding or the resources to be fully supportive. I look back at that and I know that it could have been life threatening for him.

I: *Did you say anything directly to him about what you had witnessed?*

A: *We talked about it afterwards, about how we knew it was because he was black that they pulled us over, but I don't think I had the understanding to be able to ask him the right questions about what his experience was with that.* There are phases that white people go through with our guilt and our shame and one of them is the apologising phase. During my apologising phase I messaged him and apologised to him for not having handled that better.

I: *Did he experience you as supportive in that situation?*

A: I don't know, and this is one of my best friends so it's hard to know that there was a lot more that I could have done.

I   *As an educator and therapist what is your experience of assisting healing from the trauma of racism?*

A: I love doing this work transculturally and with other white people. It's something that I inject specifically into my work with white people. In the past for me being white was an invisible normal thing, now I bring it into the room and question it. "What's going on here, we are two white people talking about this?" Because of my bio and the things that I've written on my website I get a lot of white people who are interested in looking at these narratives for themselves. I also work with a lot of immigrants and it's helping me to be the support for them that I haven't been able to be for others in the past, but not in a self-serving way, feeling like I'm writing the wrongs of the past. Now I know better, and this is what I can do today, and it helps me have a lot of honest conversations with my black and brown clients. I'm able to say, "What was that like to say to a white person?" and I can hold the discomfort of being a representative of the oppressor group

I: *Have you been supported in this by your peers, supervisors, educators, family, and in your CPD*

A: My training was largely not helpful or supportive for this, largely out of not knowing how to deal with it themselves. A lot of it has come from working with you. I've done a lot of reading, and I have been supported by my family and friends. My mom reads everything I tell her to read, and she's been helpful in reminding me to keep compassion and understanding for other white people as she's doing her own learning, specifically about missionaries and colonisers. She is understanding for the first time that those are the same thing in a lot of ways; So, my family are really on board. My first primary supervisor was a big help. He was a man of colour which was always very present in our work. With my second primary supervisor, race was not something that was brought up a lot, or that I felt supported bringing up a lot. I really struggled with her regarding gender and sexuality as well.

My current supervisor is in her 60s. She's white and she's awesome at managing this kind of work. With her, it feels like she's meeting these kinds of internal struggles with me, with compassion, so she's taking a very similar approach to you. It's nice, to be honest, on the remnants of my guilt, to not have to rely on a Black woman to do that work with me. I hope to become a supervisor like her.

I: *What did you draw on from your life experience, peer groups, studies, reading etc*

A: Like I said I've been so lucky to have grown up in a diverse bubble, where my friends and I have always been comfortable talking about religion and race and gender and sexuality.

I: *How do your intersecting identities, white, female, US, contribute to self-understanding as a white person?*

A: Being a woman is my only marginalised identity and that gives me the empathy that I need to understand how other marginalised identities rage at the oppressor group. If I were a straight, rich, cis white man I wouldn't know how that feels. I can never know what another person is feeling, but I have some understanding based on my own anger, powerlessness, fear and sadness that come because of living in a patriarchal society. I'm a white immigrant with an American passport which comes with its own layers of privilege. I've lived in Asia; I've travelled the world. In a lot of places, I stuck out like a sore thumb but not in an uncomfortable way because people bend over backwards to help you when you're white. I think the intersectional identity of being an immigrant and seeing my own privilege in that and having experienced other people's experiences of immigration, makes me very passionate about it and gives me the empathy and understanding I need to one day make that experience better for others.

I: *How does this contribute to understanding about white racism and your own hurt from anti-black racism*

A: It gives me the empathy I need to understand others and allows me to know where I may cause pain to others and to try to not perpetuate this cycle.

I: *Do you think that's an accurate statement' whiteness hurts?*

A: I'm gonna say yes and I feel uncomfortable saying it, because I think it means a lot of fear, and generations of old pain. It also hurts to see that I am part of the problem and to know that I can do all the work and do all the things, but I will never be able to do enough to change the whole system. It hurts in a lot of ways, including the guilt and shame that I'm feeling saying that to you.

I: *So, we came back to shame and that's what you were feeling at the beginning, when you saw the questions.*

A: yeah, yeah

I: *So, would you equate guilt and shame with hurt? Would you say it links to your hurt?*

A: I don't know, though guilt for me has become a good feeling. It's an uncomfortable feeling, but usually guilt means that I'm doing something that I should have done a long time ago or confronting something that I should have confronted a long time ago. It requires looking at an old wound which is sometimes painful, but I wouldn't automatically associate guilt with hurt. Shame, I don't know. something inside of me is going, "They're not the same." There is pain associated with the shame but it's not the same as hurt, but it's only a half-formed thought.

I   *That's OK, I was just extending that a little bit, to link with the question that I had originally asked as my title, because I'm thinking, you know all these things that we experienced, guilt, shame, ripples of terror, rage and in the first instance you said, 'white people are afraid'. I'm thinking what was the hurt that caused the fear in the first place, that then got in the way of feeling empathy and connection?*

A: My white guilt and white shame are 100% rooted in my religious upbringing. Which is what that whole paper was about.

End

To show some diversity of white interest in the theme of anti-black racism I present an interview with L.

I: When did you first become aware of your skin colour as a white woman?

L: I was born and brought up in a working-class area in East London, where being white was the norm. My first awareness of skin colour, and the fact that white skin seemed to be considered 'best', was in primary school where there were racist cartoons and caricatures in books, and we were made to give pennies 'for babies in Africa'. The curriculum in the 1950s taught us how we white people were 'civilisers' and what a great job we had done around the world.

I: When did you first notice whiteness and become aware of white racism? How did this feel?

L: At a personal level, probably the first inkling came when I was about ten. A young man who worked with my father had a girlfriend from Mauritius and my parents made a big thing about the fact that she was black. Her looks were commented on and there was a sense that she was different from us and 'exotic'. I knew there was something strange about the way they were talking about her, but I didn't understand it. I felt confused more than anything.

In my mid-teens, I stayed with my pen-friend in Paris, whose family were Tunisian Jews. As a white Romanian- and German-heritage Jew, I was brought up to believe that all Jews were white and Yiddish-speaking. That summer taught me that Jews can be brown and Arab speaking, with a culture totally different to mine. This time I felt angry with my parents for giving me a false sense of the world and I felt disdainful towards them.

The biggest awareness of the racism I have been 'marinated' in came when I was in my mid-twenties. I moved to Birmingham and that was the first time I had extended contact with Black people. I finally had to face huge feelings of terror and grief. I was working as an action researcher with 13–16-year-old girls who were deemed 'at risk'. I had a white colleague and an Asian colleague and at the end of the research period, the Asian woman said she would publish her findings separately, as the research framework was white-focused and inherently racist. Me, my white colleague and our white supervisor got very defensive. I felt angry and I felt it was unfair. I just wanted to argue. I remember saying I couldn't be racist as my grandparents had been murdered in the Holocaust.

After that I began to understand that there really was something I had to look at and that was the beginning of facing the fact that my ignorance and prejudice and privilege hurt Black people. I was shocked once I understood about structural racism and where I was complicit. I decided to 'change my mind' and subsequently my actions. This means things like reading and educating myself, building connections and real relationships with black people, making mistakes and working to rectify them. And noticing how limited my mind still is and how much is left to clean up.

I: Would you say that you have felt hurt by white racism?

L: I think that being white and 'marinated in racism' hurts because it denies the ability to be fully human. For me personally, some of the hurts I experience come from -

- my ignorance and what I don't know I don't know
- learning and facing the reality of the impact of racism and feeling powerless and ineffectual. The way racism operates in the mental health system and the criminal justice system
- the times I am a bystander and don't speak up or act out of fear or uncertainty or not wanting to be unpopular
- the act of being lied to and misinformed about the world, especially from people I trusted
- seeing up close how racism hurts Black people
- seeing what it costs emotionally when you can't hide or 'pass'
- making mistakes and hurting others
- my apology not being accepted

I: In what ways did you experience the hurt. Physical? emotional?

L: Any of the hurts are always visceral. I feel them in my body as tension, sometimes nausea

I: Were you able to talk about it with anyone?

L: I value being able to talk about issues with some friends, both white and black. I have a network of white peer counsellors with whom I talk and openly express the emotions I feel about racism as a white person. I think more clearly as a result and am more able to take effective action. I also do this with white people in workshops I lead on ending white racism.

L: When was the first time that you openly supported a black or brown person experiencing racism? What was this like?

L: The first time I supported someone being targeted by racism was when I was 18. I had a work placement in a children's home and every evening the owner would take the one Black child and dress him in her jewellery and scarves and make him dance and sing. He was about three years old. I knew this was wrong but I'm not sure I articulated it as racism. Though I was very scared I told my placement supervisor about it and the home was inspected and ultimately closed because of many issues of abuse.

I: How do your intersecting identities white, female, Jewish, contribute to self-understanding as a white person?

L: My family were Romanian pogrom survivors on one side and German Holocaust survivors on the other. I grew up surrounded by an unspoken relief that finally someone else was being picked on. And I was continually told the world was dangerous, that people didn't like Jews, and no-one was to be trusted. This made me feel unsafe, 'special', alone and clearly fuelled my racism.

Focusing on my oppressor material as a white person forces me out of a state of victimhood, [whether as a woman or as Jew or as a survivor of the mental health system] and expands my life as it becomes less limited by feelings of fear, superiority, shame and guilt.

Summary

Writing this chapter was not easy, because the title assumes behaviour and attitudes of members of the perpetrator group. Listening to white voices articulating their responses to questions about anti-black racism is something that I am not used to and rarely put myself forward for. I found parts of it quite painful.

My knowledge of this previously came from literature and observations of perpetrator behaviour, during training. The chapter is hinged on developing my compassion and acknowledging the hurt of white people, that steers their role in anti-black racism.

Whilst attempting a second draft, I lost the chapter. When I recovered it, I found it was corrupted. I asked for help and failed to get it represented from 'unreadable', back to the first draft. For some reason, I was forced to revisit and restart the review process. My internalised racism was rife. I discussed with my writer's support group the possibility of it being jinxed, because of the content. Thoughts that followed the incident were in the vein of, it's the theme of the chapter. Was I not supposed to write about white people in this way? Why is this important to show? How does exposing this aspect of anti-black racism support a black Empathic Approach? Which white people will share honestly their hurt, and experiences of their engagement with racism? Sharing this connection and experience has certainly been a way of demonstrating the black Empathic Approach. The chapter is about my curiosity and empathic offering to white people, so it demonstrates the book title.

Some of my early rage about abandonment by my mother got entangled with my rage about anti-black racism, and the white perpetrator group. I now see that if I can show more of myself and my own struggle with anti-black racism, I have more emotional space to develop a black Empathic Approach with white adults. This aspect of developing my compassion has become essential to forgiving perpetrators for all the oppressions that I have experienced throughout my life and forgiving myself for the ways that I have internalised and colluded with anti-black racism and hurt myself in the process. As the most challenging chapter, both lost and found, I need readers to know that the writings I wanted to avoid, that eluded me, have become essential to the black Empathic Approach and this book. An important learning for me was confirming how guilt and fear feature for white people in their responses to anti-black racism. I also noticed that my own guilt and fear contributed to the emotional roller coaster of my writing in this instance.

This chapter has been particularly challenging, in many ways. I guess the challenges are lingering within my feelings of inadequacy as a woman of colour and not directly experiencing the theme as a white person. From this most humbling place, I realised the deep introspection needed to achieve compassion and open mindedness about the hurt associated with being white. This is not something I had fully contemplated on my journey. Nevertheless, I'm realising that switching off my rage, to be more compassionate is not an easy task. It is a gradual process of revealing myself and being open to the stages of my emergence from rage. I can feel the landslide beneath me and it feels as though I could be swallowed by this territory rather than held. It is a gradual process of revealing myself and being open to the stages of my emergence from rage.

Chapter 7

Developing an appropriate gaze

The existentialist philosopher Jean-Paul Satre introduced the concept of 'the gaze' in his 1943 book, Being and Nothingness. He suggested that the act of gazing at another human being creates a subjective power difference, felt by the gazer, and by the gazed at. Consequently, the person being gazed at is perceived as an object, not as a human being.

Lacan in Bailly (2009) referred to the symbolic order, influenced by the gaze, for example, the male gaze, from which gender hierarchies and divisions emanate. He suggests that once a child has learned the rules of society, it becomes more content.

For BIPOC Individuals in predominantly white societies, this aspect of assimilation can be interfered with by colonial thinking, and a distorted gaze. Hence the evolving process of internalised racism. Lacan viewed the gaze as a powerful element of social interaction. It reveals where a person is focusing their attention, and, when directed at us, it can have a strong emotional effect. The gaze can play a role in power relations. A direct gaze can demonstrate social dominance and gaze aversion can indicate social submission.

Responses to the 'racist gaze' Kaval (2023) start at an early age. Following this, individuals respond to the type of gaze they have received, and in their attempts to identify, they build coping references and mechanisms. At the same time, if not aware, individuals raised within perpetrator groups, can be growing their rationale for racialisation and racist behaviour. This can result in hurtful behaviour towards the subjects of racism.

When I visited the Jewish Museum in Denmark, I was disturbed at seeing a display of literature showing that some antisemites in Europe, produced books for children offering a negative gaze towards Jews, as a means of their early education. Well-meaning parents who participated by obtaining this type of literature, would have played a role in coercing their young ones to stay safely distanced from Jews.

In my own situation, there was an absence of identities other than white Anglo Saxon, displayed in literature and this had a similar effect. I did not notice the distorted images of black people in the literature that I had been offered, but there was something in me that resisted this lack of an appropriate gaze, and I preferred to look at books and comics with images of animals.

DOI: 10.4324/9781003479994-8

The black Empathic Approach encourages therapists to acknowledge anti-black racism or racialised processes and expect them to name this situation as it has been described, or experienced by the client, or person seeking assistance. This is not just providing a space for them to get their experience or feelings off their chest. There is another step, which is about paying attention to the details of this process and the powerful feelings associated with the experience of anti-black racism. Once there is attention to the traumatic impact of racism, an appropriate gaze can be developed. Otherwise, the therapist may be distracted by their own defences, and their own coping skills, or internalised racism. In preparedness, this approach requires therapists to work through the hurt and trauma of racism pertaining to themselves whether they are in the subject, or the perpetrator group. Thus contributing to healing a distorted gaze.

November 2023

Another BEAP workshop has taken place, and feedback suggests that facilitators are experiencing some fear about an incident in the workshop that was clearly a perpetration of racism. We agreed that an opportunity to challenge had been missed due to internalised racism. One of the facilitators became unwell overnight with stomach upset and diarrhoea. She linked this somatic incident to severe recognition trauma. The following day when facilitators used their power to show transparency in the workshop and address the internalised incident, healing occurred, and the stomach upset ceased. I reaffirmed that we are all a work in progress and that after acknowledging the mistake and the imbalance that internalised racism had created, success in providing an appropriate gaze had been achieved.

I feel blessed that for myself, having missed out on an appropriate gaze, I eventually became a mature student and learned more about the world, my identity in the world, and other ways of being. I questioned the missing bits in my training And the Eurocentric gaze of my upbringing and education. As a result of this, I have learned to listen to myself and to others and to be responsive and encourage empowering ways.

My rage is taming, but there are certain situations where it rears its ugly head. I know I can learn from the fire in my belly and as Pinkola Estes (1996) suggests. 'Rage is a teacher'. Learning from rage is fundamental to the black Empathic Approach. I guess the framework for this approach emerged when I decided to forgive my white mother for abandoning me, and my black father for dying before he could raise me. This forgiveness culminated in an early stage of building compassion for myself and others. I believe that forgiveness plays a significant role in the development of compassion needed for conveying a black Empathic Approach.

This new way of thinking about myself and my identity as a black mixed heritage woman, entered my psyche after a Reiki treatment that had been gifted to me by a white Jewish friend. During my time of receiving divine healing energy, I had a vision of my mother. An epiphany came with the vision. I realised that the Anti-Semitism and ancestral history of the Holocaust and oppressions that my mother experienced through her connection with my late black father, had caused her to abandon me at the age of five months old. I learned later that it was possible to build my forgiveness into acceptance and understanding of the hurt that lay below. I could transform this learning into tools that have supported others in similar situations.

This epiphany was a profound moment of forgiveness and release from the angry self I believed was a normal part of my identity. Somehow through the healing hands of my white Jewish friend, I received insight that would change the future relationship with myself and others. My internal gaze had been distorted. Until that point, I had harboured a lot of anger towards white people and mistrust towards most human beings. For a third of my life, the message I had told myself was that no one could ever possibly know how to love me. This was a starting point where I could think differently about how others saw me and how I could see myself.

Offering a black Empathic Approach to support others therapeutically, requires much more than a brown skin that has experienced being abandoned, misogynoir or racialised. This ability needs to be located within self, either as a person of colour or someone embodying white privilege as a member of the perpetrator group and their association with inherited patterns of slavery and colonisation. Within the profession of psychotherapy and counselling and in recognising personal and institutional challenges of anti-black racism, therapists must make opportunities to transform the current gaze.

Until recently my gaze was highly influenced by my rage. I realise that I have mentioned rage before, but I have not written extensively about it. I have used the term 'black rage' to describe rage that arises as a result of racism. It's not rage at oneself as a black person, though some of it may emanate from internalised racism. It's not rage that has the colour black, it's rage about the injustice of white privilege and the harm that this can do to individuals and groups. This rage is not the same as everyday rage, although we are subjects of racism every day.

Rage is not something referred to in everyday language. I have heard comments such as I'm annoyed, I'm irritated, or I am angry, yet the term 'rage' has been silenced. As humans we can become triggered, infuriated and rageful. These are different levels of powerful feelings related to discontent, injustice and downright protest.

A child can be forgiven for what is often known as a tantrum and righteous indignation, a display of kicking and screaming and vitriol, to put attention on needs that may have been ignored. Sometimes adults want to shut down the raging, screaming, demanding child.

I do not remember being in that state in my early years, but I do remember, my adolescent self, slamming doors and throwing things, and the threat of being caned and punished for what was deemed to be bad behaviour. In the children's home where I was raised, the main method of discipline was making the children feel bad and being told we were sinners by using quotes from the Bible. That put a level of fear into me, and I grew up being conscious of how I might be seen if I were loud and unruly.

I have a demeanour that portrays calmness, but there have been times when I have felt murderously angry. Those close to me will know that I sometimes shout when I feel unheard, frustrated, scared, or unseen. This contradicts the silent, withdrawn, hypervigilant part of me that wants to shut my noise down, so that I am not abandoned or rejected.

There are many questions about the term 'rage', because it's not a common term. I can see why it's not used much, because rage that turns to outrage, is often interpreted as madness.

When my youngest son was very small there was often a battle between him and one of my granddaughters. They argued and fought a lot. One day I said to them I'm going to give you fifteen minutes to shout at each other. They were surprised. They used the opportunity to scream loudly at each other and say anything they wanted. After that they became friends and having used a safe place to vent their rage, the battles did not continue.

Rage can be loud. When voices are raised, the body is saying let it out. Western adults don't often allow themselves to do the shouting and raging for fear it becomes destructive, or we are seen as mad, rather than being mad at someone or something.

It is not a negative thing to feel rage in relation to racism. Yet there are punishments. The term used for Mental Health sectioning of black men seen as 'big black and dangerous' meant that their rage was often misunderstood. This led to their over representation in the UK Mental health system.

Cooper (2019) emphasises 'rage as our constant companion' P34. When we are raging there are multiple layers to express. Our rage about intergenerational features that have oppressed us in various ways, from being told how we should be, and being punished if we are not the way we should be.

Cooper goes on to suggest that we should make our rage count. Looking at it this way offers a kind of freedom to vent disagreements and heal from hurts about the way we've been treated. Once these powerful feelings are expressed through the body, by the body, outside of the body, then there is possibility for transformation and developing an appropriate gaze.

Rage shows us that we have powerful feelings that want to be expressed. Rage is an expression of injustice. Having the capacity to rage without injuring ourselves or others takes integrity and self-knowledge. White Western societies encourage us to talk about rage nicely and dampen it down, so, often we feel that we cannot wildly express it.

I looked on one day, when my other granddaughter aged two was raging in public. She knelt with her head to the ground and screamed into the concrete pavement at the top of her voice. Her mother watched and stood close to her allowing her to vent every bit of her anger until she felt calm enough to raise herself into her mother's waiting arms. This was a very impressive act of love and positive, unconditional regard. She has two small children now and two generations later, I am witness to her rational attitude to their behaviour. I see generational progress in developing an appropriate gaze, very different to how I was as a parent

I don't remember being that patient with my own children. I do remember looking around to see who was watching and a feeling of wanting to curb the shame of their loud expression and righteous indignation. My own anger as a child was either ignored or curbed with punishment and somehow, although occasionally I screamed out, I am now able to make my 'rage (in Coopers words) respectable' P 152 (2019).

Toning down rage into a respectable way of being can mean that it is not freely expressed. Therefore, how do others know what we are really feeling, or how furious we really are about a situation.

Lorde in Cooper (2019) suggests that 'women of colour in America have grown up within a Symphony of anger, at being silenced, at being unchosen, at knowing that when we survive, it is in spite of a world that takes for granted our lack of humanness, which hates our very existence outside of its service'.

Cooper (2019. PP164, 165) goes on to discuss the ways in which BPOC hold themselves together. The idea of 'respectability politics linked to rage is seen as a "rage management project"'. Respectability politics was a survival strategy in the face of massive potential for violence. A way of looking good so that we are not seen as bad and unworthy. Cooper (2019) 'This can be seen in ways that black folks often have everything in place when we dress, because many of us were dressed smartly, our hair groomed tightly and close, conformatively in tune with western modelling'. She makes an interesting observation of how the gaze can affect BPOC communities. Citing Michelle Obama's presentation in the role of first lady, and the Constant reporting of her mode of dress and her style as 'perfection' and 'respectable', that gave her credence as a black woman. It was not difficult to tell when she dressed respectively but her demeanour was not in tune with certain events'.

Cooper (2019) notes how 'black women can cuss and pray at the same time', yet this untidy venting does not attract empathic responses. On the contrary, others witnessing this phase of outrage often become terrified as though this is violence'.

The stereotype of 'angry black woman' has been used to dismiss the pain experienced by BPOC individuals. This has also been a common feature of internalised racism, and a distorted gaze, where she fears displaying her anger, in case she is labelled in this way, and her feelings are not taken seriously.

Cooper (2019. P93) quotes a phenomenon named by social scientists as 'the racial empathy gap' in which people, regardless of race, believe that black people experience less physical pain than white people. This racial empathy gap influences everything for BPOC, from harsher sentences for crimes, to differential prescribing practices for pain medication, the birth mortality rate, poorer health outcomes and overrepresentation in the mental health system.

This is why there is a need to specifically address a black Empathic Approach to psychotherapy. It may just be a way of addressing the racial empathy gap, and a way to consider an alternative to toning down and expecting 'respectable rage'.

Cooper (2019) recognises the delicate intersectional situation of black women carrying too much emotional and ancestral baggage, that can add to explosions of rage.

Cooper (2019. P167) 'It is difficult for rage and respectability to exist in the same place. Suppressed rage will cause us to accept gratuitous violence as a necessary evil. Expressed rage offers us an opportunity to do better'. For example, the Black Lives Matter movement was born out of rage about police brutality against black people.

I often express a few expletives while getting the rage out of my system, however, my respectable rage shows up in my writing and teaching.

My father addressed a distorted gaze in one of his letters. He stated that he and my mother were from the two most hated nations. Her family fled the pogroms and came to Western Europe where Holocaust survivors soothed the experience of a negative gaze by building relationships with African and Caribbean post slavery survivors. I am from a Catholic and Jewish background, and I was raised as an Anglican to continue the legacy of hiding Jews to keep them safe.

Somewhere far away from that children's home my grandma lit shabbat candles on a Friday at sundown and made kneidel soup. So don't ask me if I am Jewish just because the synagogues are full of white people.

We are not all the same and our diversity makes us special. How would you talk to your three-year-old about life, her ancestors and their rich cultural background? What if you had been raised by people who ignored this?

Here are some questions and comments that I would like to have voiced about the gaze to my white carers. Why did you find my hair difficult to manage and why did you not learn about ways of caring for Afro hair and brown skin?

It was difficult enough coping with period pains and being born different to my African and Caribbean peers. In school they seemed to accept me, and they shared their ways of talking, their music and being black. That teacher Mrs Brian used to shout at the black girls and tell them to behave differently as they are 'not in Jamaica now'. I witnessed this in secondary school. She seemed to be full of contempt towards them and I felt it.

Because I speak like you, this does not mean I am like you. In Trinidad, they asked me why I tried to speak like them, in Ghana they called me 'white lady'.

You made me feel that my father was not my father, and my mother was not my mother because I did not resemble them. You cannot define me by who my parents were.

I was the brown girl in the ring encircled by questions about who I am. Am I black? Am I white or in between? I was asked if I am half-caste. I have now eliminated this slavery term from my vocabulary. Of course, it was painful and I had to try and forget my bewildered self and find an appropriate gaze.

Kaval (2023) P52

Unconscious racism in everyday living impinges silently on the psyche, affecting feelings of self-worth and the cumulative impact can even create feelings of profound confusion in what you think, feel and who you are, when the sense of self has been colonised by the racist gaze of another. This type of assault on the capacity for freedom of thought is often caught up with feelings of weakness, shame and humiliation, which invites and necessitates a type of therapeutic engagement that can bear witness, empathise and articulate an inner agony, that cannot be voiced, in the hope that this will enable the victim of racism to face the unnameable and protect the self from the subtle and overt ravages of racism in everyday life.

Kaval (2023) offers examples of the 'Racist Gaze', this being an impingement on the psyche that can affect us every day and lower self-esteem. He refers to this phenomenon as an 'agonising, often unspeakable, assault on the psyche'.

This damaging and confusing state can create an unstable identity experience for individuals. A confused identity can disturb responses to an experience of racism, and contribute to a distorted gaze, thus deflecting an empathic, compassionate response and creating defences, such as rage and anger. In which case, support for healing the traumatic impact of racism would be lessened.

We may ask ourselves, is it possible to evolve from such a deep internalised experience of the racialised self? In writing this book I am living in hope of the possibility that a revolution in personal gaze begins with awareness and a determination to haul oneself out of the mire, into the light and create new ways of thinking and being about the effect of anti-black racism.

Offering empathy that embraces thoughts and feelings about personal experiences of racism can be an intense and enduring experience. However, this would assist in the development of an appropriate gaze. It would be futile to focus solely on the negativity and traumatic impact of racism, so an appropriate gaze would also be empowering and affirming of cultural origins.

In a recent discussion, a black male contact declared that he did not see black and white, and that racism does not affect him. He went on to share his concerns about Asians leading the country and he came out with a familiar diatribe about having experienced more racism from his own people. Although he says he understands racism. I cannot expect empathy from him, so I question our acquaintance. If he is confused about racism and freely blames people of colour, how can I trust that he would support me in my work? I feel that someone who has numbed themselves to the pain of racism and his own identity cannot be a useful ally to me or provide safety. Incongruence is not supportive of a black Empathic Approach to psychotherapy. A person with a distorted gaze cannot be fully aware and confident about how they may listen to or support another person who may be harbouring confusion about their identity, or experiencing the trauma of racism. They may offer inappropriate responses, judgmental ideas and misunderstand or disconnect, to defend their own identity. They may distance themselves from unbearable experiences, even with those close to them. Sadly, two negatives do not make a positive.

Being Jewish does not automatically mean I can be empathic regarding the hurt of anti-black racism. I can, however, if I am aware and have experienced an appropriate gaze, as a Jewish person of colour, use this experience as an empathic response to experiences of racism and the effect of white privilege.

In her talk on 'Being White in a Racialised society' Ryde (7th Marian Fry lectures, 2009), discusses self-reflection and interrogation of whiteness, white privilege and fragility. Ryde says she doesn't often think about being white (white privilege). She started her PhD from the premise of exploring her own whiteness and regarding her class position. She wanted to find out what it was like to be black. She refers to white people who call themselves black to align with the oppressed. This is not empathic. It is an indictment of modes of anti-black racism, and can serve to dismiss the reality of white privilege.

It stands to reason that many BPOC individuals who have not experienced a reflective same identity, may not have experienced a black Empathic Approach and consequently not experienced an appropriate gaze. This may also mean that many who have trained in Eurocentric disciplines may not be tuned in to a black Empathic Approach. In addition to personal upbringing and coping skills, this culminates in a lack of training and expectation of this approach to racialised experience.

Ryde (2009), recommends a non-dual, intersubjective, co-created experience in the therapy space, thus finding truth through understanding and acknowledging the diversity of cultural values, rather than judging the other person. Seeing reality through diverse experiences, rather than splitting off into good and bad. BEAP is in fact, more nuanced than this. If all this is going on, then empathy towards subjects of racism is not given a full opportunity to arise and be expressed.

She talks about the narcissistic ideal of being 'white'. Her language and enquiry as a white woman are impressive, but she backs up her perspectives with Eurocentric ideals, concepts and approaches. I am concerned that this way of seeing, interpreting and presenting ideas can also co-create a revolving circle. Ryde left the audience with the question. Do you get a chance to discuss being white? I would add to that, do you get a chance to discuss being black, mixed heritage, or a person of colour? The gestalt experience, so that this is an opportunity to explore racialised identities.

Ryde (2009) felt guilt throughout her research process. She grappled with the context of shame and how we respond to colonialism and systemised racism. She uses the term 'unconscious racism' to examine her thoughts about the intellectual ability of black people as opposed to white people. This is where we must be cautious about white people writing about anti-black racism from their own experience. I believe we need to be conscious about our responses and how their experiences, though valuable, may not be wholly empathic or supportive to subjects of anti-black racism. They just are what they are in terms of the white experience, and due to lack of hundreds of years of lived experience, have a different perspective on the subjects of racism.

Anti-black racism is political, personal and psychological. I clearly remember an occasion when I found my voice against bullying and racism.

As an adult, struggling to feed my children, I became an Avon lady. Poverty and single parenthood forced me to trundle from door to door in my local neighbourhood. Selling products to raise money to feed my children. There was a point in my selling career, where I realised that black women were my main customers, yet I could not fathom how makeup presented by Avon Cosmetics, was not created for their skin tones. Although I was an agent for the company, I took courage to enquire about this lack of sensitivity to BPOC skins. I wrote a letter that was ignored, so I withdrew my services from Avon. This act of resilience showed me that no matter how tough my life seemed, no matter how much I needed the money and flexibility of earning, if this company were not hearing my voice and I was slipping into the role as an agent of oppression I needed to take a stand.

I researched ways to articulate, explore and create alternatives that mutually support, process and attend to powerful feelings that racism evokes. And this became a key component of the 'black Empathic Approach' to Psychotherapy. It is a tool that, combined with an appropriate gaze, can bring about transformation in attitudes and behaviours regarding the impact of racism.

There is no blueprint for this training because it requires leaders in the field to see the need for change in attitude from the top down. A sculptor friend once said to me that to rebuild something you first have to break it down. Builders, artists and creators know the importance of taking courage to break something down and rebuild it with tougher, more appropriate and durable materials. This is the context for which I am proposing a black Empathic Approach.

Having worked with statutory and voluntary organisations on change with regards to institutional racism, it has become clear where the power for change lies. Investment in breaking down white privilege, and developing an appropriate gaze has to be seen as a priority in systemic change. This is fundamental to class systems that maintain poverty, ignorance and inadequate pathways to environmental and human involvement in the manifestation of cultural confidence.

It takes a village to raise a child, therefore the villagers must all play a part. We have seen generational changes that show how language, attitude and healthy, non-judgmental approaches to personal development can elevate self-esteem. Out of this, leadership that promotes inclusion and eliminates oppression can emerge. But there must be role modelling and mirroring that promotes gateway's to breaking down the effect of white supremacy, genocide, and internalised racism, and rebuild systems that do not collude with white Eurocentric, colonial, anti-black perspectives.

Summary

In therapy training we are taught about reflecting, paraphrasing, mirroring and providing a gaze that supports the other to see themselves. We are taught to create a knowing that reflects self-understanding and new ways of being, that build congruence, self-love, positive life relationships, equality and confidence.

Teaching that reflects monocultural Eurocentric perspectives, and those who did not grow with awareness of the limitations of their training, were disenfranchised via academic and sociocultural learning. These conditions coexisted alongside white privilege and internalised racism. They undermined emergence from cultural and racialised existing preconditions of slavery and colonialism. They did not allow space to explore and elevate individuals and their respective groups to reckon with the damage caused by these discourses, and therefore willingness to work through the trauma imposed was not measured or supported. This caused silence within training and therapy provision. The need for willingness to emerge from this silence is fundamental to a black Empathic Approach and an 'appropriate gaze'.

Notes on world impact of Anti black racism; genocide, imperialism, colonialism- 43 genocides occurred between 1956 and 2016, across the African continent, resulting in about 50 million deaths. The UNHCR estimated that a further 50 million had been displaced by such episodes of violence up to 2008. Since April 15, 2023, 8.2 million people have been displaced by the conflict: more than 6.5 million have been forced to move within Sudan and around 2 million fled to neighbouring countries, notably Chad (36%) and South Sudan (31%).16 April 2024.

https://reliefweb.int/report/sudan/5-million-people-sudan-experiencing-emergency-levels-hunger-after-year-conflict?>

Anti-blackness is about making sure we stay as victims in our internalised oppression and internalised genocide. Millions of people have been displaced and starving in Sudan, Kenya, Nigeria, Congo, Ethiopia, coupled with fighting and killing each other for resources. All resources that support the Western world come from Africa. For example, Titanium, pillaged, stolen and colonised in Africa, due to widespread, anti-black racism and internalised racism and not speaking up. BPOC are grieving for our ancestral homelands, and our communities of origin. We are led to believe that Africa is poor, instead of the truth, that it is victimised and colonised. We are not responsible for having these ideas installed into our minds. We need to learn how to recognise them and interrupt them in all areas, including education.

The route to an appropriate gaze.

1 Notice how anti-blackness shows up in your thinking and in your life
2 Notice how you think about and respond to black people, black culture, black bodies. Notice, assault on black bodies, black beauty, black worth, black power. Notice where there is a desire not to be seen as black, or desired as black. i.e., skin bleaching, European speaking, Notice attitudes toward black presenting.

Notice attitudes, beliefs, understandings, and behaviours reflecting all of the above. This quote by Steve Biko says it all.

https://shoppeblack.us/top-steve-biko-quotes/

REF 'I'm going to be me as I am, and you can beat me or jail me or even kill me, but I'm not going to be what you want me to be'.

Chapter 8

Unburied and undried tears

We often use the term low self-esteem. Being low or feeling low is a consequence of feeling powerless to change a situation or feelings associated with it. Grief underneath these feelings may be deep inside, but unburied, because harbouring these conditions influences our coping skills and the behaviours we may use to hide or mask our true feelings. In highlighting these behaviours, I am embracing the possibility for change.

In 'Zong and the Black Outdoors' (2017) Phillips talks about being transplanted, as many local flora and fauna in the Caribbean. She passed the Poui tree, on her way to school, in Trinidad, yet was not being taught about the tree. They were taught about daffodils instead. She used the term 'Hydra headed beast of colonialism'. In other words, not having a mother tongue and experiencing lack of inner safety, s a child expressing loudly her grief and joy,

Phillip's mother would tell her 'Don't be so loud, you sound like a Jammette'. (*women on the street*) linked to stigmatising of Spiritual Baptists, previously known as Shouter Baptist. I am using the term 'unburied' to refer to the silencing of inner expression and identity. Curbing and internalising grief and rage is a primary source of internalised anti-black racism that therapists need to turn their attention to.

Tobago 2021

I am sitting in a favourite place where I often have breakfast and watch the ocean. I have been to a yoga class. My body is feeling stretched, my breathing is even, and I am at peace. My tranquillity is intercepted by the voice of a white European known to me. She calls out 'hello'. I look up and we greet each other in a post Covid way. She exclaims. 'Tobagonians are primitive'. I am appalled at her ignorance. She, being someone who has visited the island for 20 years and absorbed the cultural nuances of black life here. Racism is around every corner I think to myself. This is significant for the unburied.

I reply, wanting to say 'I find that racist', but my internalised racism kicks in. I compose myself and politely say 'that is not very nice'. I am silenced. She continues to exert her white privilege. She tells me that as a Dentist she knows science

DOI: 10.4324/9781003479994-9

and barks on about the percentage of Tobagonian citizens refusing to take the COVID vaccination. I am clear she has no idea about the cultural back story to this issue. She is ignorant to her blatant racism, and I do not want to be involved in blaxsplaining in any shape or form. I silenced myself, and made my anger respectable, looking away from her.

She walks away. I am left with mixed feelings, hurt, anger and the impression that from her Ivory tower and looking down her Western nose, she feels it's OK to say this to me as a light skinned black person. I am much lighter than many Tobagonians. The wound is deep, and my internalised racism is triggered. I feel grief for myself and my ancestors. I don't expect to be in my ancestral home and experience this blatant anti-black racism. I realise that my perspective is naïve, and I momentarily forgot that colonised thinking and white supremacy is smeared all over the world. I cannot hide from the anti- black racism that I have experienced all my life, and it is chipping away at my identity.

As an essential feature of communicating a black Empathic Approach, therapists need to be aware of how we can numb ourselves or act numb in our observations and responses, when anti-black racism has taken place, or when racism is prevalent in the lives of others.

At that moment I had become a victim of racism, and I needed to reclaim my power. Being a victim of racism is the point at which racism becomes internalised. My identity has become thwarted. I allowed myself to be thrown overboard with my black African heritage Tobagonian peers. I did not fight to stay on board, because of my fear of consequences and the power of white privilege. My response was not a deliberate choice, it was a conditioned response to lack of safety and an immediate need to protect my skin.

I have always been a subject of racism because it is in my life, and I am a member of the subject group by nature of my skin colour and being raised within Eurocentric paradigms; However, in knowing the point at which I descend into victimhood and become asphyxiated by the tide, I gain knowledge of the importance of empowering myself and noticing that I am not drowned yet, I am numb and trying to keep at bay my recognition trauma.

Awareness of our cognitive dissonance and how individuals may be seen when we act numb is a vital part of the black Empathic Approach. This is a point of accepting these powerful feelings in the underbelly of internalised racism, where sorrow is awakened and attacks on the BPOC identity becomes apparent.

Grief

My undried tears and grief stayed within me, silenced, attached to the loss of my parents, and significant others. I had never been part of the village or a community display of grief for loved ones, until I visited my homeland. My father passed away before I could utter his name, I knew very little about death and dying, except that my tears were undried. I was silently grieving as a child for unknown ancestors and my fragmented family. Opportunity to talk about the loss of my loved ones has been rare, but I have always held them in my heart.

Age nineteen, I arrived at my mother's funeral and found that the casket was nailed down and a silent group of people, called family, not showing emotions were present. They appeared gagged and bound as though physical and emotionally restricted from movement and self-expression. They were my family, separated from me in my early days. And there were others who I assume were my mother's relations. It was as though I was watching a movie.

I now feel blessed and humbled that I've had many endearing experiences of saying goodbye to relatives and friends about to leave the earth. I can only describe these experiences as enriching and spiritually humbling.

I watched my Trinidadian sister decline from a stalwart, church going woman who managed her diabetes, too timid skin and bone, taking her amputated body and confused brain to the grave. I returned to visit her in Trinidad every year during the long period of her dementia and inability to function without assistance. I learned to be unconditional and kind-hearted to her when I recognised her terror as she hallucinated and saw things that I couldn't see, that threatened her safety. When she batted away food that was offered to her. When she would strike out a fist at her enduring husband while he attempted to help her. Those final days with her were a blessing. I could see that she was fading, breath labouring as she tried to gallantly hold on to life. Before she sighed her final resting breath. I gave her permission to leave and reminded her that she is loved.

Having met her for the first time in my mid-thirties, I remember being impressed that a grown woman, in her late fifties, could express her emotions easily and cry every time I left her and returned to London. It was easy for her to display grief, and her tears were symbolic of the freedom to grieve. The ability to allow my tears was something we shared. Our difference was that she cried with love and longing for our closeness. I cried when feeling hurt, frustrated and alone. My undried tears about separation from my family stayed locked inside me for many years.

Support from the re-evaluation co counselling community gave me permission to loudly share and express my rage and grief. I also attended several grief rituals led by Sobunfo and Malidoma Some. These rituals offered me divine ancestral connection with the deep heritage of collective African grief, and my tamed experience in the Western world. There is power in writing through my undried tears. I am now clearly aware that every time I cried as a child and as an adult, my body was cleansing a lifetime of grief, internalised racism, misogyny, sexism, identity confusion and sorrow for myself and others, as a mother and therapist.

I grieve for all the clients who wanted to talk about their lives as black people, the cruelties and challenges of being seen as not enough, as less than. Those who were beaten, demeaned and treated as less than human, those not feeling loved enough or loved too much and those striving to be better than, when they are good enough. Those who like me, were misunderstood and misrepresented, gaslit and starved of affection and warmth in their young lives. Those who felt the ugliest and the blackest, the family Cinderella, perceived as the only one and the least intelligent. Those loved for what they could do, not who they were. The ones that felt abandoned, like me, and lost in a world that doesn't value their family origins and the way they inherited speech patterns that were straightened out in elocution lessons. Confused by immigration and assimilation and ignored by teachers, elders and such like. Clients seek someone to mirror who they really are and offer hope for some inner security. A comforting truth that might give them hope that they are ok, worthy of social recognition and emotional love and acceptance. Worthy of having their tears tenderly dried. Worthy of burial and a loving goodbye on their way to eternity.

This is my thought process about a black Empathic Approach from within me and applied to me, having found myself being unburied. I am aware that my grief is coming from my black self and all that goes with my intersecting identities, including the loss of close connection with my white Jewish mother, my black African heritage father and my mixed heritage siblings.

Living in Tobago has helped me strengthen my black self. I'm guessing that a black Empathic Approach would have come to me directly from my siblings if I had been raised with them, but to this day, we have not spent enough time together to foster our collective grief in a natural way. Maybe we would have supported each other or fought with each other, called names, jeered and somehow pulled each other through the mire of identity confusion and searching, that can be a part of growing up black, mixed heritage.

Moving through these thoughts about my own emotional and spiritual growth, I arrive inside a process that provokes a wish to encourage others to lean into what I have called 'recognition trauma', and engage with the powerful feelings evoked by internalising, silencing, and noticing that anti-black racism affects all of us. There is a choice for those who want to emerge from colonised thinking, and a false sense of ourselves, to become who we really are on the spectrum of life as we grow and get to know ourselves more deeply.

When I am in conversation with people who I deem to be insensitive or not aware, I may come across as powerful and coping, a feature of the 'strong black woman' demeanour. I have found myself asking them to consider me as a person that hurts, by saying 'I am not made of stone'. I'm sure this is a feature in the lives of many other BPOC individuals. This perspective of black women is part and parcel of Eurocentric, unconscious racist thinking and is to be considered in a black Empathic Approach.

In Zong, Phillips (2017) 'The Sea Has No Back Door' the author expresses the horrific scene of slaves who felt the sea was preferable to finishing the journey, on the slave ships. The alternative was being stuck with thousands of persons' excreta and vomit. They became the ungrieved and the unburied. Dredging on the surf and tossed on the waves. Portraying the fragmented echoes of wailing and weeping through the turbulence and across the ocean. Shuddering, drowning, dying, floating, decomposing. Unnamed, drowning, flooded, choking, praying, chanting, dying, suffocating, singing, naming. Reflecting the dismembered, rotting, abandoned bones, rejected, swept away, selective drowning. Flailing, swimming, asphyxiated, transposed, disintegrated, diseased. Jumped or flung overboard cargo.

This was the lament of the fragmented souls of slaves, lost in transatlantic middle passage crossings, who never arrived and were never permitted to achieve freedom on dry land. Those who floated in the ocean with the scars of the master's whip, washed over by salty waves, away to unknown shores. Taken from loved ones and communities with no burial rights. Their disintegrated bodies were carried by the waves of no farewell, and no burial. Strewn across the ocean and not returned. Grief Symbolic of this inhuman, transgenerational history can be witnessed in present day attitudes and behaviours. Though not comparable, in propagating the term 'unburied', I am concerned with dead but not buried, symbolic of unexpressed grief. Persons denied the rituals of expressing grief and letting go of the physical and spiritual remains of a death or loss of identity due to anti-black racism. Loss of the precious and personal is not the same as letting go of the pain of abandonment and rejection.

Alleyne (2022. P73) refers to this phenomenon as 'hauntings' that are present in both white and black peoples' psyche.

'For black people, hauntings are experienced as attacks on their racial identity. For white people the ever-present terror of retribution for the sins of the colonial past. Perhaps spooking the white conscience and leaving fear in the white collective unconscious. As in white fright of the black other.'

'A guilt complex emanating from repetitive historical guilt that manifests as hyper alertness to perceived danger from a black presence'. A black Empathic Approach in this context can be seen as a personal, political and psychological, acknowledgement of the terror, abandonment and grief lying deep within descendant's psyches and the need for a place to grieve for the hurt of our history.

Arriving at Elmina Castle in Ghana, there was a sense of doom and the lingering pong of incarcerated slaves. I witnessed the 'Door of No Return' through which abused and rejected slaves were cast down a chute into the sea, as worthless garbage. Schultz (2003), writes that by the 18th century, up to 30,000 slaves passed through the 'Door of No Return' each year. It was not difficult to imagine the stench of brutalised bodies and the agony of this hellish journey. What could have been worse, to stay or go?

In that time and place, I experienced a deep empathic connection to physical, emotional and spiritual brutality; their story merged with my story.

In our history. In world history. The curse of human cruelty. The destruction of life by other humans, evidenced in slavery, in ethnic cleansing and annihilation created by war weapons. So, what is it to be human? What is humility? What is humanness? I am rageful about the damage to humankind. Sitting here writing about it, I make a tiny crack in the hard-edged shell that holds down the compassion needed to harness the thing I call a black Empathic Approach.

This poem was created after my journey to Ghana

Poem Elmina Castle prayer.
Christmas in Ghana (Mckenzie-Mavinga 2003)

ARRIVAL

Tequila sky
melted stress
delayed flight
Katoka Terminal
in sight

Akwaaba
A word in Twi
meaning welcome
Akwaaba mamma
They say

An Afro-European
with dollars, pounds
baggage carriers
fight for custom
I purchase hands

I don't see holly
only tree lights
sold in boxes
on roadside
Tataquashie market
rosewood giraffes
Merry Christmas
one Santa cap

My son Nyameche
negotiates a sale
They say
I have good price
Ashanti images
Carry Africa's spirit
for loved ones

Nyameche names
A carved hippo

Kwesi
His Trini-African friend

AWAKENING

customary greeting
welcoming water
A shared vessel
thirst quenched
the soul libates
Djembe, Djembe
raising a tender beat
over coconut palms

we breathe
In excelsis deo
Glory hallelujah
Sahara swirl

They witness
my non-belonging
coded confusion
speak from your heart
they say
what to tell my children
when I go be with them

To belong
Not belong
Language limited
alien
in forefather's land
strange yet familiar
Nkrumah, Dubois,
Padmore, my Dad
campaigned
against fragmentation

Remote village
rights of passage
bush bath
three wishes
Ancestors

connection
The see-er points
Go to 'Fishponds',
Queen mother
to your
Fulani people

CONNECTION

My heart speaks
God's cock-a-doodle-doo
oven baked dawn
red soil footprints

I'm curious
about Akosombo
dam re-settlement
Misplaced
eighty thousand
Lower Volta residents

What have I in common?
'Look at us' they say
hungry children
traffic light beggars
outstretched hands
I am a guilty tourist
not buying from
the speechless man

Kente weavers,
plantain sellers
beg me for sale
want my things
for themselves

They yearn for England
say they like the cold
'Give us your address Mama
take us to your soil'

DISCONNECTION

I know nothing
about war,
about famine
about disease
poverty, sightless,
speechless,
limbs, on wheels
on crutches

Biting in my face,
stinging my heart
I want to bat them
like flies
get away,
out of my sight

INTOLERANCE

pointing fingers
clay villages
women pissing
in the street
speaking from my heart
the Shell, 'Mobil Mart'
an Internet shop
tinned beans
Cadbury's chocolate
bring relief
my exit to Europe

strange vomiting night
the gut of indifference
through my Western eyes
bile of Africa ejected
duty free distaste
devastation

As Africa's fragile economy
my body requires help
from those away
those returned
those at home
Babies crying,

mosquitoes feasting
'Good Morning'
says Echo
the night watchman
'I bring fan for cooling'
Our languages clash
we talk with arms and eyes

KAKUM RESERVE

Rainforest bridge
my soul suspended
each step swaying
reminds me to breath
I fear
don't look down
no safety net
the jungle beneath

Door of No return
unburied ancestral cargo
A wailing ocean
Walls remember
Rape and pillage

A stench
like no other
histories burden
rocks my equilibrium
grief shakes my body
crushed and broken
I crumbled
Sistas catch me
I am humbled

PRAYER
Almighty Cape Coast
Creator of love
of universe
I ask your blessings,
your love, your greatness
wash away the blood,
mucous, urine, faeces,

vomit and terror
of enslaved ancestors

Let scars be healed
cleanse repercussions
let past despicable acts
not prevent our liberation
Cleanse away bitterness,
de-pollute our energies
let them not be diffused
nor convoluted

Let us live in harmony.
guide us, deliver us
heal the wounds
that make us take up arms
Let us not re-enslave.
let us be our brilliance
the best we can
to kinship families
forever.
Amen

ACCEPTANCE

I see
women pounding fu fu yam
fish cleaning
for coal pot
millet soaking
for Banku meal
tired scrubbing boards
infants hang sleepily
behind each bend
Each sway cradles
to the rhythm
of dirty linen

Men stretched on benches,
under moonlit kerosene lamps
the dawn coconut vendor
becomes twilight taxi driver
currency expensive

in Sterling
Cedes are cheap

REJECTION

Brown Barbie girls
too worse for liquor
sport flattened hair
they call me 'white lady'
Not nigger

I speak from my heart
I want my familiar
ready to return
to cold walls
stony faces
hidden whiteness
be black, brown
be in between

Have a few pounds
not millions of Cedes
be Afro familiar

but
I will not hear
Akwaaba
or
Welcome home
Mama

Undried tears decompose, smell rancid, and expose a lack of care and attention. This state symbolically represents neglect, shrivelling options, and lack of action toward the possibility of annihilation. There is a stark powerlessness in this position.

I know I am not enslaved, yet still I sometimes feel as though I am at sea. Tossing around without a rudder, or an anchor. Unsure of where I am heading and what to hold on to. That's how I am feeling as I write this chapter. It's almost as though I am lost, offshore, afloat and untethered. At the mercy of an unforgiving ocean. At this point I need to reign in my compassion for self. So, I turn to my notes, my reading and the tools of support that I know of. I realise, It's not true. I am not rudderless, or without anchor. I am recovering from a weekend of pain. A symptom of my illness. Something that whilst I am alive, I can overcome. I need to remember that I am not in this alone. If I am stuck, I can ask for help and break the silence of tossing around in the waves and the turbulence of my aloneness.

The last 3 days I have been in a vortex of pain, bewilderment of a kind that goes with writing. I am fully aware of the diverse undulating waves of a writer's block, but I do not remember experiencing anything so physically and deeply blocking as this. On reflection, I feel like I became deeply locked into ancestral pain that could not be expressed in words. That I did not know how to express in any shape or form. That had me deciding not to fight it, but to rest and do nothing, but doing nothing is not an option Andrews (2013) for me, as a powerful independent woman.

It takes a lot to knock me down and to decide not to fight feelings. Once I became aware of trying to deny the pain and helplessness that I was experiencing, I surrendered. Someone watching over me would have told me so, but I struggled alone. Only God and the ancestors and divine Reiki energy were watching over me and helping me through these times when I needed to trust, and I do. Allowing this experience to transform this chapter has reminded me that I am not writing alone.

This morning, I came out of the mire, like a phoenix rising. I experienced physical pain in the early hours and calmed it with a rare dosage of paracetamol and my early morning Reiki practice. Coming out of a dream about losing one of my children, not in a way of them dying but in cutting loose from me, has given me another sense of my grieving as a single parent. In other words, my children have flown the nest. They have their own lives, and I have mine. No matter what has interfered with our close bonds, the ties are never cut.

Coming to terms with physical and emotional distance while finding our lives can be like an emotional rollercoaster. I have revisited this part of the journey many times in my dreams and often wake up feeling bereft, unsure of my single elderhood and needing to make physical or emotional contact as a form of reassurance.

I have a meeting scheduled with someone who has chosen to support me with my legacy work. I am reassured that this person who has come forward and is actively showing their passion for my work has got my back. They are helping me push this work forward. This reinforces the need for me to remember I am no longer abandoned and no longer rejected. I am loved. The physical and emotional pain of the last three days has subsided, and I am ready for this challenge again. I can harness my compassion. Now I return to the question of rage transforming to forgiveness and compassion, necessary for a black Empathic Approach.

I confer with Cooper's writing (2019) when she talks about having used her anger to help others, but I have also learned how to control it. She encourages readers with a comment about champion tennis players, the sisters. Cooper (2019. P6)

> The sisters have figured out how to corral all that power into precise serves and shots that are nearly unmatched. They have created this kind of alchemy that uses their physical strength and strategic prowess on the court, together with all the racial slurs and insults they have endured over the years, to create something that looks magical to the rest of us.

Yes, we have seen this on the tennis courts, on football pitches, in the media, in the film industry and in the wonders of all the survivors, whose ancestors were unburied.

During one of my early visits to Trinidad, local people asked me why I tried to speak like them.(I must have been code switching) In Ghana they called me 'white lady'. Sometimes I was a bit of a Chameleon, but my skin could not blend in.

Why did you confuse me by acting dumb and making me feel that my father was not my father, and my mother was not my mother, because I did not resemble them. I refuse to be defined by who my parents are. In other words, the grief and discombobulation were not laid to rest. As a grown woman my grieving and burial rights have been self-made. Expressed in safe places where others have joined together in ceremony and ritual about our heritages and black empowerment.

Tobago January 2024

I woke up this morning at about six thirty. The sun was rising and there was a slight breeze. The atmosphere was already warm. I pulled on my jogging pants, a pair of trainers and a T-shirt and embarked on my first walk of the week. As I walked up and down the undulating hills of Sou Sou lands, I felt alive. Being in the elements is my happy place. A dog lay basking on the warm concrete. A hen was demonstrating to her newly born chicks, how to drink from the water running down into the gutter from the house above. A little boy was bringing the sheep up the hill to their grazing point. Another child was feeding the chickens outside her door. I could hear voices in the distance and the occasional vehicle starting up for the journey to work. As I placed one foot in front of the other, in my ancestral heaven, I felt at peace. I turned a corner and was greeted by a local couple taking their morning stroll. The man called out to me, "how is the snow?" It seemed they knew something about me that I didn't know they knew. This familiarity is one of the ways that makes me feel at home here. We don't know each other yet we know. I replied,' that "I had left the snow behind". He called back that they had also left before the rough winter weather. Within an hour, I arrive home, take a shower and some breakfast and settle to my writing. Being able to appreciate the warmth, acknowledgement and caring of my people reminds me that compassion is in me.

In the book of forgiving, Rev Desmond Tutu (2015) suggests that, when we tell our story we heal. It is a chance for freedom and forgiveness is giving up hoping that the past was different. I am learning to give up disappointment attached to relationships and systems that do not serve me.

In therapy there is an expectation of naming the hurt and telling our stories, to repair a broken past and build a new future. All this means building self-compassion, and building confidence in our identities, whoever we are. First, we need to forgive ourselves for self-blaming and for cutting off wonder and beauty. For the harshness that we have harboured and projected onto others. The lack of self-care, flagellation, remonstration and quarantining feelings. For deeming ourselves unworthy of love and deep friendships. Second, we need to welcome ourselves, say our names and love every part of our fears and feelings until we become one with them. Third, we need to harness hope and be charitable to ourselves and others. Be open to positivity and humble connections. Give up past and present disappointments and embrace change wholeheartedly. I see this as an aspect of drying our tears.

Years ago, I went to a grief ritual with Malidome Some. It was held in Greenwich Park in South London. Together with several other people, we chanted and named loved ones whose physical beings we wanted to release from the earth and our longing for what they represented to us. The ritual was symbolic of releasing our personal challenges, dead things and giving them permission to move on out, therefore releasing ourselves for new life. A few years later, I joined a group led by Malidome's wife Sobonfu. To the sound of African drumming, we dug a pit and took turns to express loudly into the pit what emotions and useless life patterns no longer served us. There was screaming, wailing and weeping. We were encouraged to express our rage at those who had dishonoured, abused and done hurtful things to us. A lot of dirt went into the pit, and this was symbolic of letting go and burying oppressive things we had been carrying deep inside us. Then we lit a fire in the pit, and cremated those past relics that no longer served us. I see this as an aspect of burying the unburied.

I learned from engaging in these ceremonies, that there is something spiritual in the practical aspects of ritual. In doing this we can cleanse our psyche. We link the divine with our beings and open our hearts to do the work of our ancestors. There is a lot to be said for group rituals that cleanse and witness our progress. When I worked with women impacted by violence in relationships. I placed food at the centre of our meetings, food to nourish them and we burnt paper with their expressed hurt and rage written on it. These efforts to release and create symbolic burying of harboured negativity gave them permission to seek less harmful ways to cleanse their unexpressed thoughts and feelings and allow their tears.

Summary

In this chapter, I referred to the 'unburied', symbolic of unexpressed burdens, whether they be dead or alive, or buried alive. These unexpressed burdens often link with unprocessed traumatic experiences such as racism. Harbouring them is akin to internalised oppression and the mental, spiritual and emotional damage that anti- black racism can do.

A tendency to go numb rather than express feelings means that our feelings have been deadened. Dead but not buried because certain faces, places, smells and situations remind us of past traumatic or hurtful experiences that can bring these feelings to the surface.

I use the term trauma to identify the deep hurt that racism instils in its subjects and perpetrators. A black Empathic Approach recognises this impact of racism on individuals. It is a way of providing a route to compassionate healing. Humans become retraumatised by certain frightening, abusive happenings, so I believe that it is important to partake in periodic cleansing rituals to eliminate the oppressions we internalise, that can undermine our healing processes and our identities. We may be well practised at disassociating and deflecting from these triggers, until our minds and bodies experience a critical mass and prompt opportunities to release the trauma and grief stored inside.

Lee Lawrence (in his courageous memorial to his Mother Cherry Groce, shot and paralysed, by UK police) (2020. P268) wrote,

> it's not enough to think things will just happen; to keep applying the pressure to make sure. None of this is easy. None of this is a quick fix. But in a year when statues to slave traders are torn down and a memorial to my Mum is put up, now feels as good a time as any to make a start.

This is a prime example of celebrating and releasing, rather than burying

Rage, hurt, silenced feelings, rejection abandonment, undermining, slavery, terror, subservience, self-flagellation, attacks, code switching and skin bleaching, pigmentocracy, white privilege and fragility associated with fear, guilt, shame, rage, denial, vulnerability, misdemeanours, mistakes, secrets, disgust, agony, powerlessness, weakness, to name but a few, are some of the unprocessed feelings and heartaches associated with being unburied and having undried tears. I suggest that these powerful feelings lay in the underbelly of 'recognition trauma'. This is a route to presenting a black Empathic Approach.

Chapter 9

Reclaiming the minds we never lost

Tobago 2024

A visitor to the island told me she had been attacked by three dogs whilst walking. After that, she became afraid to walk on her own in the area where she was attacked. When BPOC individuals experience an attack of anti-black racism, whether it be physical or emotional, this can cause similar trauma.

The woman was not mentally unwell, she had been terrified. It is clear that the mental and emotional toll of an attack often gets ignored, causing trauma to build in the human system. The trauma is often unnoticed until a change in behaviour and worrying symptoms occur. Many BPOC individuals shut down after a racist attack. This silencing is a common coping mechanism.

I had an indelible experience as a toddler, turning confusion and abandonment in on myself. Left alone in the children's home, I remember tearing out my hair and tossing it over the edge of the cot onto the floor. Apparently, when this was discovered, I was taken to a doctor, who suggested that I needed consistent care from one individual, instead of being passed from hand to hand by a group of strangers who were the white care workers in the children's home where I was living. I was taken on a long holiday by Auntie Nancy, a kind-hearted staff member who offered some initial bonding. These days she would have been viewed as a key worker and my condition identified as a mental health problem. From a distance, I can see this as a form of early self-harm aimed at my natty black hair.

As I entered adolescence, I was subjected to the staff frequently cutting my hair because it was viewed as difficult to manage. I was saturated in humiliation at an early age, and I experienced intersectional oppression emerging from internalised racism, early childhood misogyny, sexual abuse and ridicule at school, because of my mixed black, white identity. These experiences were compounded with internalised Anti-Semitism and abandonment. The Barbican Mission to the Jews, where I lived, was established at the end of World War two. They wanted to convert the children into Christians. They were missionaries who themselves had been converted and then rescued children separated from their parents due to the pogroms and being sent on the Kindertransport from Europe. My fate was sealed

DOI: 10.4324/9781003479994-10

in a version of Christianity, that propagated white privilege and the ten command-
ments. Throughout most of my young life I experienced the threat of hellfire and
damnation if I did not conform, and my young life was void of intimate emotional
connection and touch. I managed to comfort myself with food and I harboured
mistrust of the adults around me, who seemed emotionally disconnected. What
I have now learned about human connectedness and the need for trust, touch and
intimacy has given me insight into the usefulness of empathy in human connection.

Renowned traditional Psychoanalysts, Bowlby, Winnicott and other Eurocentric
theorists presented views about 'attachment' and 'separation' in early childhood
and established psychological theories that challenge ideas of child welfare and
adult responses based on levels of connection.

These theories contributed to stereotypical approaches to adult psychotherapy,
and they did not address detachment and belonging that included loss of heritage
and cultural community and the rejecting influences of anti-black racism.

Rogers in Clarke (2022. P15) tells us that 'Subjective processing can be emotionally compromised by practitioners biases and prejudices, leading to distortions
in client understanding and strains in the therapeutic relationship'. On the other
hand, an objective empathic modality may also be a barrier to effective treatment
when a counsellor or a therapist assumes impersonal and objective ways of relating
to a client.

'Subjective empathy enables a practitioner to vicariously experience what it is
like to be a client for a momentary period of time' (Clarke 2022. P15). 'Through
a resonating process a counsellor or therapist activates internal capacities of identification, imagination, intuition and embodiment when reacting to the immediate
experiencing of a client'. It is this area of identification that therapists must be wary
of, in terms of challenges that may arise in the use of a black Empathic Approach.

Unlike generic empathic responses, therapists need to be aware of their ability
to slip into a campaigning mode or silence. In this mode, strong feelings about
racism and the inability to manage their own trauma can trip the therapist into the
role of wanting to rescue, do for, influence, or jump on a bandwagon full of rage
and revenge about a client's experience of racism. These powerful feelings, in other
words, the therapist's own 'recognition trauma' can seduce them out of the counsellor role and flatten their empathic responses to racism.

Clarke (2022) supports the context of identification whilst connecting with a
client's experience as a transitory process. An essential prerequisite to separation
from the client and stepping back and allowing them to reclaim their power.

Recovering from the impact of racism means surviving the historical and
intergenerational grief that goes with assimilation, whether voluntary or coerced.
This requires an authentic will to humble ourselves to the process and impact
of colonised thinking and behaviours such as name changing, code switching,
skin lightening, hair straightening, voluntary servitude and harbouring a 'slave
mentality'.

Our minds are, and always were, robust enough to manage these elements of
psychological warfare, once there is a decision to work therapeutically in this way

and harness appropriate support for empowerment. I believe that a black Empathic Approach can contribute to helping others reclaim the minds, they thought they had lost and the minds some people were afraid of losing. There are ways that BPOC people have been gaslit, when challenging anti-black racism, or when attempting to find a safe space to unravel their powerful internalised feelings linked to racist experiences. The result of these responses has created confusion and discombobulation, sometimes leading individuals to believe they are losing their minds. This concerning state of mind needs to be greeted with an appropriate gaze, that supports empowerment to strengthen mental health and connect with the dilemmas of internalising racism.

Postnatal depression is a diagnosis given to forms of depression experienced after childbirth. The mental health system accepts this diagnosis as reality, because there is evidence that a real baby has been born.

I see that trauma associated with experiences of anti-black racism is real. After a racist attack, or repeated covert experiences of racism that undermine individual self-concept, personal assistance to think clearly about well-being and ways of coping and building self-esteem may be needed. As racism is not always overt, therapists need to check their belief systems and the ways that they can gaslight or undermine experiences of anti-black racism and, therefore, add to a client's fear of losing their mind.

Furthermore, when a BPOC individual enters the Mental Health System, due to an experience that may appear to be other than racism, it is vital that consideration is given to how anti-black racism may also have impacted their self-esteem and coping skills. This is a black Empathic Approach.

When I worked in the African Caribbean Mental Health Association in Brixton, I became aware that a familiar skin tone and a feeling of home from home, created a level of safety for clients. They experienced this as empathy from people who looked like them. There were also times when imbalance seeped into staff relational well-being, caused by systemic racism that crept into behaviour. At times, shadism and class differences divided us. As a BPOC group, we were unified in purpose, yet at the same time, there were difficult interpersonal relationships, due to skin tone and behavioural attitudes. I call this the effect of internalised racism. Staffing levels and funding issues meant that opportunities to work through these oppressive forces were limited. This showed that we also needed a black Empathic Approach to leadership, that could help staff develop relationships, more conducive to our well-being and the well-being of our BPOC clients.

If staff displayed behaviour, that appeared unsupportive or not empathic, clients experienced nothing more than an extension of ways they had been treated in the Mental Health System and other statutory organisations.

An example of this is the time when a client bit the receptionist's finger because she pointed in her face, instructing her to leave the premises. The client was demanding to see me when I wasn't there. I never saw her again and I guessed that she was restrained, and frog marched back to the hospital. The staff group trundled along in a kind of numbness that silenced and divided us.

Incidents of suicide, neglect and misdemeanour that occurred within the mental health system and were brought to our attention, were not explored. There was no significant responsibility for moving these systems on and attending to our own collective internalised racism and recognition trauma.

Trained therapists can experience internalised subservience to colonised thinking systems that encourage binary conditioning towards clients. An unlearning process that addresses internalised racism is needed. This can seem scary. Students may feel threatened that their professional certification will be jeopardised if they appear rebellious against these systems.

Trained therapists may fear that their membership with professional bodies will be revoked, if they ask for more, or turn towards alternative ways of thinking. There is a fear that they may be labelled disruptive, and therefore unruly, as slaves who did not cooperate. The mental health system has too often been the next port of call for some individuals who could not cope with these confused teachings, that have coerced their empathic abilities, to not see, hear or act towards the damage that anti-black racism can cause.

The saying 'have you lost your mind?' or 'are you losing your mind?', or any other label that goes with not feeling balanced or somehow being off the colonial grid, suggests a form of rebellion or resistance to systems that cannot cope with or decipher the hurt and pain of psychological gagging (silencing) and the ways many have been taught conformity.

I have a Rasta friend who always reminds me that I am free. I also have women friends and peers who offer me good ideas; they have great minds, and they inspire me to develop my own ideas and not give up. Some therapists trained specifically in a black Empathic Approach who know what this means, can offer an appropriate gaze. Lorde (2007) suggests that, in sharing the pain and grief of racism, we give and take, to keep sane, as this journey requires radical self-care.

The musician Curtis Mayfield expressed feelings and fears of isolation, internalised racism and madness in his song *'Hard Times'* (Hard Times was written by Curtis Mayfield and was first released by Baby Huey in 1971). A decade after Martin Luther King's speech. 'I had a dream'. This was a period in history when the impact of anti-black racism was becoming unsilenced. In the song, Mayfield presents an image of 'cold' eyes staring at him. People all around in 'fear', and denial, not seeming to want him. Mirroring himself as some kind of creature having fits. He is afraid to come outside of his house. Though filled with love, he is afraid they will hurt his pride. He plays the part expected of him and pulls the blinds, so he won't see them seeing him. He repeats the mantra of 'hard times', where there is no love to be found, in the 'crazy town'. He wants to see familiar faces and meet others including his brothers, but he is surprised that they are corrupt and want to hurt him. These are haunting words that explain the mental suffering that can occur with isolation and mental ill health.

The song reminds me of a visit I made to Tooting Bec Psychiatric hospital in the nineties. I spoke to an Indian woman sitting on her bed. I could see the terror in her eyes. She took a while to respond to my invitation to talk. She asked me if I could bring her slippers. I took that to mean that she wanted to walk away from her bed and be somewhere else. Anywhere away from the madness and chaos of her mind and the restrictions of the hospital ward. The next paragraph describes how humans have become victims of robotic responses, such as 'AI' that can further isolate us.

Tobago 2024

On waking this morning, I have a blank slate. I wanted to prepare myself for embarking on this chapter. I've received an email about a financial situation that needs clarification. Ok, I thought to myself I can spend time evaluating the situation and deal with it efficiently within a short time, then proceed with my writing. I was wrong. I could not locate the documents on my desktop, that would help me with the said problem. I could not get onto my banking app, no matter how hard and creatively I tried. I became frustrated and I paused to eat some breakfast to fill the gnawing gap in my stomach. That did not work. Later I communicated with the bank's chat facility. That did not help, because I was being directed towards a digital Q&A, when I needed a human being to discuss with and help me understand. I thought about my wish to not engage with facts, figures and mathematics, because this is one of my pet hates. An area in my life where I feel inadequate.

My inadequacy does not stem from an inability to learn maths, or lack of being able to work with figures. It stems from childhood low self-esteem and insecurity about my confidence in this subject at school. I could add, subtract and divide by rote, but I would not raise my hand to answer questions of any sort. I was the brown girl from the children's home who did not know anything about life. My inferiority arose from feelings of being the odd one out. The one with no family support or encouragement. She was not aware that she had a good mind and was equally capable of learning anything and retaining confidence in her ability. She kept herself silent in the classroom and no one noticed her need for more information, clarity and attention.

This is my story, and I continue to reclaim my mind, knowing that the possibilities of continuing to learn and develop confidence are endless. This sacred right is one that every human being should be afforded.

During my morning of AI discombobulation, my son interrupted with a call from his hospital bed. An unusual morning call. He wanted me to listen to his extreme frustration at not having his discomfort and pain attended to throughout the night. He was being told. There is a nursing shortage. He feels bullied and neglected when the nurses ignore him and make him wait for hours to be cleaned up, and his pain attended to. This is dehumanising and repetitive on days when the ward is overloaded. He named all the oppressions that he was aware were contributing to his in-patient and disability neglect. I have never heard him so clear about what could be going on. Instead of approaching this from a victim stance, he named racism and several other oppressions in the pecking order of hospital life. I listened, knowing that not only was his physical health in jeopardy, but he was aware that his mental health was declining.

'I can't breathe he said' and no one is helping me. Being starkly aware of that statement echoing through our communities, I stilled myself and with tears in my eyes, I put my own distress aside and gave him my full attention. The implications of that phrase hit me like a ton of bricks. A black Empathic Approach was in demand. He felt pushed to his limits. He needed me to assure him that his mind was intact. While we talked, a nurse appeared at his bedside, and he told me she was preparing to clean him up. He called back twenty minutes later and told me that the job was done. His face looked more relaxed, and he was comfortable enough to chat about the cold meals he had been receiving, because it took ages for anyone to feed him. This was a lighter conversation.

When his anxiety was soothed, I tried to get back to my accounts, get them out of the way and return to my writing. It didn't work. I was feeling stressed, and I needed to breathe myself. I needed a hug, but there was no one there. At times like this I question whether I'm losing my own mind. My compulsive independence kicked in and I thought of people who I might call for support, but it was just a thought, and I struggled on.

Yesterday was Valentine's and before retiring, I joined an online meditation session about self-love. I turned to what I knew would best help me to breathe. I cleansed my space using sage, incense and Reiki energy and did some simple yoga, guided by an online app. This helped me to calm down. Life goes on and takes its peaks and turns. I want to write from this vulnerable place that I'm in today and be transparent about my own mental health and my own fears about going crazy. I'm in my yoga pants and vest sitting on the balcony in the breeze and getting on with my writing at last. The financial task that distracted me from my morning can wait and I am alive and following my passion.

The 26th of January 2023 was the first day of freedom for my first middle child. After a year on probation following three months in jail, he became free to work and travel as he pleases. His last few years have been troubled, having been homeless and struggling to maintain work, good health and his own sense of well-being. I had defended my black son from bullying in primary school, but the teachers didn't seem to get what I was seeing, and his fighting back was just merely seen as aggression. I did not feel heard or supported by them. He was the child artist who wanted to be an architect, whose white female fourth form teacher wanted him to become an athlete. In his defence as a young black man, I had challenged his teacher about trying to channel my child into a stereotypical vocation, typically assumed by a racist educational system. Things went downhill after that.

Instead of embarking on A level arts his career ended abruptly. He left school prematurely and I felt helpless as a single unsupported mother, knowing he had been bullied by the police on his way home from school and by grown white men in public spaces. He left home and started his career in the gym pumping iron, to make his image bigger so other men would not mess with him. His subsequent body dysmorphia and engagement with substitute fathers and a man's world led him to ketamine and other mind-altering substances intended to help big him up and numb his mind to the pain of his fatherless world and the racism. My biggest fear is that he will continue to be treated as big black and bad. Also, that those who cannot see his vulnerability, will continue emasculating him.

August 2024

Yesterday I visited my injured son in the hospital. It had been several months since we saw each other in person. His health is improving, yet there is a way that he remains incarcerated. He has come a long way after being paralysed from the neck down. The three broken vertebrae in his spine are healing. He prides in sharing that he got through ten months without surgery. For some reason, by the time he arrived in hospital it was too late and the injuries too complicated to operate on.

Having survived that leg of his journey, he is now able to operate the hospital bed with the electronic controls. He can stretch towards the bedside table and get the things that he needs. He can feed himself. He no longer uses a catheter but is still not in full control of his bowels. He is being assisted by the physiotherapy team and they can help him stand and motivate him to use his legs.

He gives me permission to open the blind. I view from the fourth floor the building works going on below. It is a Saturday evening and quiet from the drilling and pumping.

I put my shame and embarrassment about meeting a security guard outside of his room, away. His addiction to ketamine has put him in trouble again. He is open about his use of this self-medication, which he believes is assisting his recovery. He knows I am not happy about this, but I accept that this is one way he feels fully in charge of his well-being.

My compassion is challenged as we connect. For the first time in our life, he begins to share some details of his adolescent experience of being bullied. I have been elevated from the position of observer, to mutually sharing experiences he had previously kept from me. For many years he had silenced himself as a young black boy. Contact with his father was intermittent, yet he had contact with him that I was unaware of and gained advice from him about how to manage his experience of incessant bullying.

Many years had passed, without him feeling able to share the stories with me, his mother. My limited knowledge of his life had led me to believe that his experience of being bullied, began in primary school, and was ignored by the teachers, who saw him, at that young innocent age, as big, black and bad, in their complaints to me about his concerning behaviour.

He shared with me that in secondary school, the black girls bullied him, because of the eczema, scarring on his skin. It carried on, and he relived stories about defending himself from further bullying by the boys throughout his school life. He was advised by his father to never lose a fight. His motivation was supported by skills he learned in Taekwondo and jiu jitsu.

As he shared the story, I witnessed his grief and unburied tears as he shed his teenage experiences into my safe hands. I am challenged to notice another level of my compassion towards my grown son of forty-eight years, and some learning about his story as a young man. Whilst he continues to talk, I am challenged to keep listening and give all my attention to the hidden bits of his story that I was unaware of.

Observing his vulnerable state, gave me new insights about my compassion towards him as a black man. The depth to which I become aware of how I am affected, by being raised without my own black father has become more apparent, and I realise there is so much more to my own vulnerability and places where I can be more open to others. A doorway that may assist my developing compassion, has been opened.

Compassion requires sensitivity, kindness and calmness. I would add to the mix creative thinking, courage, congruence and clarity, as essential ingredients for nurturing self-love where rage, blame and guilt may be harbouring. I have just experienced the duality and essence of a black Empathic Approach.

My daughter's experience was the first time I felt redundant as a mother having lost another child to the binaries of a racist patriarchal system. (Section 27 of the mental Health Act, this time.) Keeping my own sanity at this time of confusion and being outside of this new phase in her life was a great challenge. I felt helpless. I guess that's how she felt too. I knew they were harder on black people in the mental health system. I struggled to maintain my composure as her mother. It was a painful realisation that as a trained and experienced Psychotherapist I could not help. I felt as though I had failed her because I could not help her to feel balanced and clear about what really happened. I do not know the full story. The antipsychotic injections rendered her to a zombie-like state and her magical dreams disappeared.

The reality was that my daughter was locked inside, and I was locked outside, and we were all in this crazy dynamic together and rendered helpless by the system. I missed my daughter and yearned for a connection with the bright, intelligent, creative left-handed child that I had raised. The next few years she slowly came back to me. I got a glimpse of the eight-year-old who would sing at the top of her voice, to her heart's delight wherever she was, and had no restrictions to her self-expression.

One day in her early school life I had been summoned to see her teacher. He described a scenario where she had asked him for some scissors that she could use with her left hand, as clearly it was difficult to manage with standard right-handed scissors. The teacher had seen her as a troublemaker because since that unresolved incident she had been trying to get the attention of the other children by becoming a bit of a comedian and disrupting the class. This showed me how easily creativity and difference can be seen as deviant and disabling.

When she was released from her incarceration, she remained under the liquid cosh Risperidone. The medication dulled her senses and made her feel she had nothing to offer the world. She said she felt nothing, and her survival was now dependent on an antipsychotic injection that she was subjected to monthly, till today, due to her continued refusal to take oral medication. Her resistance was strong, demonstrating her power of decision making and that she wanted to be in control.

I wrote this poem in 2013 after an outing with my daughter when she came out of the hospital.

Liquid Cosh (Mckenzie-Mavinga 2013)
(Refuge poem)
She strolls forward
in a trance
I on the outside
Its confusing
Isolation set in

Cheeks full
Lips pursed
Brow creased
Looking ahead
To what

An occasional glimpse
A momentary goal
She can do it
But when
When it's over

I am blocked
She sees it
Outside looking in
Inside can't emerge
I remain on the edges

Trying to keep pace
Curiously listening
Allowed in sometimes
I stay here waiting

Long silences
Sometimes stony
not hostile though

Once she laughed
My heart smiled
connection is there

Somewhere
She came from me
I want her back here

Sometimes
we look out
I look at her
Then we sink away
She is gone again
Nothing to say

She names it
DEPRESSION

Can't function well
Each day a new
Getting through
All it is for now
Be patient
You came from me
I will come for you

Two out of my four children had been caught in the system. The other two have quietly managed their grief and distress. I cannot predict how long they may survive in a world that slowly tortures you because of your skin colour and gender.

My children are parents and grandparents, and I wonder what stories their descendants will hear and how they will manage their own mental health and their responses to anti-black racism and intersecting oppressions.

This heartbreak has been a closed secret. An unresolved dilemma in my own personal development. These troubling times as a single parent of four, have been a mammoth achievement. I became stronger, prouder and more resilient, to overcome my guilt as a struggling parent, professional, and black woman. I am still a work in progress, striving to model unity, and congruent compassionate connection with my children, family and friends. The road is long, and each day is another step towards being a facilitator of my own destiny and a model for my children, grandchildren, and great-grandchildren all sixteen of them. I guess this secret is my shame, unaccounted for, unreasonable and a painful mark on my history. Looking back, I feel a degree of shame in telling the stories of my children, the story of being a mother feeling helpless in the situation of their mental health. I believe that shame is an element of mental ill health, and I also believe that sharing concerns about mental health is a way of healing.

I have put my embarrassment on the page, to encourage others to tell their stories. Mental health silence adds to the abnormal ways we think about mental health. Being a therapist, trained to work with the mind and body, I have come to believe that what we deem to be abnormal is often a normal response to abnormal life situations. If the sufferer is BPOC, there are additional considerations, such as experiences of anti-black racism, internalised racism, systemic racism and ways of coping.

I believe depression forms from accumulated oppression, and what we do with our oppressions. If therapists could just understand the levels at which we internalise our intersecting oppressions, presenting empathy might be easier.

For myself, I continue to feel rage at systems of oppression, and I work on harnessing my compassion and self-care, and growing it bigger than the rage. Maybe one day I will achieve the right balance.

Empathy incorporates feelings, reflections and context. It can be relational, yet integrative. Clarke (2022)

> While widely recognised among a range of therapeutic traditions as a core condition in successful treatment practice, empathy is too often taken for granted or marginalised due to contemporary demands for efficiency and client symptom relief. Carl Rogers' urgent call to the field to view empathy as an attitude or as a way of being of the practitioner, has largely gone unheeded outside of his person-centred approach.

Clarke (2022. P1) suggests that 'the internal functioning and deliberative reasoning of counsellors and therapists are often overlooked or neglected as significant capacities for empathically understanding clients in relational contexts'.

An experience at Broadmoor Hospital

> Orville Blackwood was a Jamaican-born British man, age 31, whose death at Broadmoor Hospital on 28 August 1991, following the administration of large doses of antipsychotic medications, resulted in wide media coverage after an inquiry into the circumstances surrounding his death were deemed to be accidental.
>
> (Wikipedia 1993)

Not long before his death, I visited him at Broadmoor hospital. My aim was to offer an 'appropriate gaze' and a 'black Empathic Approach'.

An Asian psychiatrist had asked me to discuss the possibility of therapeutic work with him. I sat with him, and we talked amiably about his experiences. And the way he was being viewed by staff. I then attended a team meeting with him, where he was not being given a chance to explain himself. Instead, the coercive voice of a white male psychiatrist was asking him to agree that he had 'a problem with authority'. He said, 'You have a problem with authority, don't you?' I found this tone to a grown black man racist and intolerable. It did not surprise me that he reacted to the attitudes of the staff.

The opportunity to work with Orville was sabotaged, when I heard a week later that he had died. The inquiry after his death stated that he had experienced heart failure due to excessive restraint and antipsychotic medication. He was the third black patient, after Michael Martin and Joseph Watts, to die under similar circumstances at the hospital within seven years. The news reports were headed 'Big black and Dangerous'. In other words, too scary to reason with, in a human way. That incident stayed with me, and I fear for my children.

In the Orville Blackwood case, it is clear that he was subject to racism and emasculation as a black man, having first been placed in prison several times, and finally, culminating in a secure institution, and seen as a risk to society and himself. There are many unanswered questions. At what point does resistance to white supremacy become a danger to society, with the possibility of harming oneself? It is essential to integrate ways of thriving and forever self-care, given the punitive nature of anti-black racism. After all, what is the point in not moving on from survival mode? Empathic understanding that includes an attunement to the pain and relief from the trauma of systemic and personal anti-black racism is key to rebuilding mental health.

Knowledge and compassion about elements of mental health that racism may exacerbate are essential to integrate ways of thriving and forever self-care, given the punitive nature of anti-black racism. After all, what is the point in not moving on from survival mode. Empathic understanding that includes an attunement to the pain and relief from the trauma of systemic and personal anti-black racism is key to rebuilding mental health.

For example, misrepresentation of distress related to racism. This includes not being believed, experiences of racism not taken seriously, low recovery expectation and misdiagnosis, due to the therapist's lack of work on their own processes to do with racism and its many intersecting features.

Acceptance of anti-black racism as a feature of sociocultural, systemic oppression and intersecting oppression must be held, for a black Empathic Approach to function. Individuals impacted by racism are often aware of their ways of coping, and the ways they have been coerced into responding politely or appearing not to respond. This aspect of human behaviour mitigates their ability and willingness to reflect and explore where their minds have been compromised and messed with. Where denial, gaslighting and undermining of experience have happened. Where they have felt as though a form of paranoia has settled into their minds and where they have blamed themselves and internalised racism as a way of coping. The fact of the matter is that they may not have lost their minds. Their minds may have become under functioning because of compressing thoughts and feelings about racism and other intersecting oppressions. There is no one-point plan to assist individuals in reclaiming their minds.

On relaying this story, I think about my son lying in hospital courtesy of Metropolitan Police having broken his neck. I reflect on similar stories. The stories his father told me about police harassment as a young person arriving in the UK in the early sixties. The intergenerational context of these experiences is stark.

Tobago 2024

On a local beach with a friend, we are confronted by an elderly white man. He had hired a hut with a group of his people. The shade under the almond trees was fully occupied by cruise ship passengers emptied onto the island that day. Having located a space, shadowed by the hut, we decided to place our seating. The man proceeded to inform us that he had claimed the territory in the shade, outside of the hut and that he would expect us to move later when the sun came on that side, and he was ready to sit there. We notice that his people we're already sitting outside of the hut under an almond tree, a distance away from us. We challenged him about commandeering the space inside the hut, surrounding the hut and in addition, under the almond tree. We told him we were not going to move under his instruction. This was a public space, in the heart of our ancestral home. The words came out 'I am fed up with this pomp and glory stuff'. In discussion with my friend, we agreed that he felt it was OK to address us in this way because we were two black women. He then went away, and we witnessed him speaking to a member of the security staff. I watched him gesticulating and pointing his finger whilst giving an account of what had just happened. The security staff, a local black man, promptly approached us and tried to explain, whilst supporting the visitor's perspective. We refused to move and told him we were witnessing a white man getting his way and being oppressive. The security staff accused us of being racist. We had the vocabulary and awareness to see what had happened. The incident marred our day, because although we laughed it off to alleviate our distress, it stayed with us. I am aware that the incident is still inside me and that is why I'm writing about it.

An everyday experience of racism such as this can be difficult to navigate internally. Therefore, it is important to consider that a black Empathic Approach can speculate that living in colonised communities we continue to be impacted by Anti-black racism and internalised racism.

Once the psyche is imposed on by these deeply oppressive experiences, it can be difficult to exorcise the pain from body, mind and spirit. In the end, we have each other as black women, as friends and having mutual experience of misogynoir, white privilege and internalised racism. The incident happened yesterday, and it is still with me. Out in the racist jungle, I was traumatised, and I question whether I want to be with my white friends that evening. Over the last twenty-four hours I have been fighting to stabilise my mind. I can tell the experience had a powerfully retraumatising impact. Another layer of racism has entered my mind, and I am determined not to lose my mind. Recording it here is one way of gaining emotional respite, capturing it outside of my body and knowing that I am not alone.

Sometimes I am vitriolic when a racist incident rears its ugly head. I can usually identify these incidents quite clearly and I must think about self-preservation and my health, in order to temper my feelings and maintain my own sanity.

The transgenerational portrayal of rage in the story of 'Beloved' Morrison (1987) depicts a tormented soul and slave legacy. The script was inspired by the true story of Margaret Garner, who, in one soul-chilling moment, *killed* her own daughter rather than return her to the horrors of slavery. The question remains, did she lose her mind or was this an act of sanity, based on her deep connection and empathy in knowing what the child was likely to suffer at the hands of the colonisers.

Reading the story presented a challenge, but watching the film helped me to understand the level of rage stirred by the transgenerational pain and torment of anti-black racism.

March 2024 Tobago

Friends in the UK are sending me videos about the protest and support for Diane Abbott on the heinous misogynoir and anti-black racism that yet again she is experiencing. The threat to her mental health and the mental health of her followers and other black women leaders in the country is huge. Tears are streaming down my face as I listen to the reports and as I watch the people in Hackney shouting their rage and demanding that she should be honoured and those racist representatives in the government be made accountable.

Shame on those who are burying their heads in the sand and shame on those who are too arrogant and bigoted to apologise and admit to their racism and violent threats. Shame on those racist gas lighters. I am sick of this racist, misogynistic nonsense. I have grandchildren living in Diane Abbot's constituency, Hackney and family in other parts of London and the UK. How will this affect their lives and their children's lives, and my children's and my grandchildren's lives and the lives of all children growing up in racist Britain?

My rage is tangible, my empathy is personal and political, and my heart is broken for leaders such as Diane Abbott who are continuously subjected to the projections of racism. I notice the experts being interviewed on the news are people of colour and I want change, but it is slow and painful. As a black woman, I feel wounded. I feel helpless, yet the power of my empathy is strong. I am spiritually with those who came out last night to protest on Diane Abbott's behalf to give her voice space and to demonstrate that she is not alone.

Our minds are tested every time we are lashed by the trauma of racism, and we struggle to maintain our equilibrium. There is little hope for this poison to be curtailed enough for a breathing space to be maintained, and healing for our communities. What do we say to our children? How can we prepare them to protect their minds from the continuous onslaught of bigotry and anti-black racism?

Our compassion must remain an element of the empathy we can offer to assist in reclaiming our minds, each time we are injured by the continuous onslaught of hatred towards our communities and individuals leading them.

I did not want to engage with racism today. I want to believe what is going on in Britain and the world is not affecting me. I want to pretend it's a bad dream and it will go away, but it's seared into my mind and body. I am sick and broken hearted at the extent to which humans can hurt and damage each other. Today I am distracted but I had to put this on the page as an example of what is important in this scenario, we call life. I shall spend some time with a blank canvas and allow the ancestors to help me express the deep, contrasting and confusing feelings within my body and mind.

As a child I cried a lot, I grieved for my lost family, but mostly in silence. I believe my silence was about not knowing a place where I could let go and be comforted. My expression of anger was mostly loud and physical. I slammed doors, threw things about the place and shouted, but there was no one to talk to and share my grief with. My expression of powerful feelings was not met with empathy. These true feelings were met with punishment, and I was silenced. As a young adult I did not have the tools to expect support and comfort.

*My teenage addiction to sugar was one of the most comforting behaviours that remains with me to this day. I am wiser about sugar addictions and its link with slavery and the commercialisation of sugar cane, sweets, alcohol and other forms of self-medication and self-harm, due to anxiety and stress. I have diabetes in my family, and I am aware how chronic diseases are widespread in black communities and how int*ernalised rage contributes to mental ill health.

For example: Diabetes prevalence in Black groups is up to three times higher than in the white population and they have higher mortality from diabetes; they also have a higher risk of hypertension and stroke. (The health of people from ethnic minority groups in England 17 May 2023.)

Summary

This chapter highlights some painful experiences and contributors to mental ill health and fears about losing our minds. It was not easy to show some of my own family experiences, but I wanted readers to see from the inside what it is like to be living the story while writing it. I have conveyed the theme of this chapter by using some of my own experiences. I want to show readers that many BPOC individuals feel as though they are living on the edge. We cope with enormous burdens that impinge on our everyday lives and threaten our well-being. It is clear that the trauma of racism is not just skin deep. Our souls are threatened by this dilemma. As I lived this chapter, I experienced the shakiness of my own life as a black woman, as a therapist, as a mother. I care deeply about the collective minds of the BPOC community, yet sometimes I feel helpless and unable.

The stories in this chapter are real, including those that have touched my life and continue to be urgent, in the sense of clearing up the mess of anti-black racism. Whilst being fully present and paying attention to my own mind during this work, I've had to be aware of now, and accept one day at a time. This chapter is a mere drop in the ocean in terms of addressing the mental health of our communities. As the environment of psychotherapy takes on progressive areas of concern, I hope that a black Empathic Approach will be taken on board, when approaching the dilemmas of anti-black racism and mental health.

Chapter 10

Black women and self-care

April 2023

Yesterday was a point in my life where I felt as though I had been wrenched back to 1994. During that phase of my life, I took a quantum leap into my identity as a black woman, acting against racism and misogyny. I seized the opportunity to work with a mixed female group of trainers presenting anti racist/anti sexist workshops to the police, fire brigade and other statutory organisations. Some of the work was gruelling as the trainer's faced resistance and defensiveness from staff who had been recruited onto the training mandatorily as part of a commitment to bring awareness into their predominantly white teams and the institutions they represented. I call this sheep dipping. The work became challenging caused by resistance to address ways of changing attitudes. Even more challenging was some of the rigid responses, from within the groups. Being in the majority, white men in positions of power, alongside white women, held the key to change.

I felt fear and my intersecting internalised racism and internalised sexism were triggered throughout the experience. Although supported by another black woman and a white woman, my impostor syndrome and voicelessness were strongly challenged. I sometimes felt powerless against a particular kind of resistance from white men and collusiveness of white women. Although there were a minority of participants who appreciated and grasped the context of anti-racism and anti-sexism, I felt left with toxic energy that was difficult to shake off.

My rage was on the surface throughout this phase of putting energy into training that felt incomplete. On reflection, my responsibility was to use my own therapy to work through early experiences of bullying and sexual abuse by white boys in the children's home. These experiences had passed unnoticed, unchallenged and unsupported. Therefore, just as I had coped with the racism, I had internalised the trauma of my abusive childhood experiences. Another task was to liberate myself from the baggage of being a survivor of domestic violence. Thirdly, having lost my father and not being raised by suitable male role models, I needed to learn about what life is like for men, especially as I have sons and grandsons.

DOI: 10.4324/9781003479994-11

Having come a long way in developing my compassion, I realise these elements as essential to a black Empathic Approach when working with gender diversity. Mckenzie-Mavinga in discussion with Grant (2023. P149)

> The benefit of working across gender is twofold. I am challenged to be assertive in getting my needs met as a black female therapist. I am also challenged to articulate my awareness of male oppression and ways that you might repress your needs as a black male therapist. I have women's concerns as well as being black, and I have experienced racism. This creates intersectional oppression.

I am aware of how the history of emasculation can operate to undermine the men in our lives. In particular, black males. This can get in the way of listening to their life stories and finding ways to support them without being in servitude. Having grown up with white women and the disconnection of being different and othered, there was a need for me to become more conscious of my role in undermining their power and ability to take charge, without constantly being saved or done for. I am realising that compassion towards black men means knowing that acknowledging their power and resourcefulness is key to building confidence in themselves and in the women around them. It is rare to see women openly challenging each other about how we communicate with men, and about men. A kind of male gender bashing happens when women generalise about men. We often forget that men are good people, who have been conditioned to do bad things to women, because of their own hurts. Women hurt each other and the men in their lives, because they have unresolved hurts caused by less evolved men. A black Empathic Approach can acknowledge and address these hurts and notice where internalised misogyny contributes to disempowerment and lack of self-care.

I often feel helpless in finding a vocabulary that displays my wish to know, accept and elevate men. This aspect of women's empowerment was not addressed in my training. I am aware of the way patriarchy conditions men for war, killing others or elevating themselves to alpha status, to participate in decimating land and communities, whilst internalising the trauma and pain of these actions. I can only assume that in Western societies, this functioning adds to the systemized gender void. Our lives are built on attack and defence systems. A small proportion of men take time to listen to our differences and the type of care needed for both parties to nurture themselves enough to value support, empowerment and self-care, that culminates in an appropriate gaze.

Because of our marginalisation in the feminist movement, strength and resilience as BPOC, women, have been marginalised. Hooks (1996) suggests that white feminism has failed to address the importance of gender and class as an intersection with racism, and these oppressions have been viewed as separate items.

There is a collusive discourse that ripples through the lives of BPOC women. The feminist movement has been liberating yet damaging to our relationships. Whilst empowering us, giving licence to undermine the black man, rather than uplift them. During slavery, black women were used to soothe black men. The soothing of black men has been perpetrated in some areas of the world, where the matriarch is she who runs the house and brings in the income that supports her man, whilst accepting subservience to his needs and the care of his children and extended family. Black women are known to become overwhelmed by the multiple roles and multi-tasking that we do. Often, our burdens go unnoticed, and we are not listened to and appreciated enough. We turn to each other for comfort and validation, and reminders of self-care. Patterns of servitude and overwork become normalised, and the challenge and support needed to love ourselves completely is limited.

In the community where I live in Tobago, I've heard young black men stating a preference for white European women, because they prefer someone who has access to greater financial resources and is less upset by the challenge and expect-ation of their misogynistic projections and dependency.

A lot of attention should be given to these themes. They arise from absent or inadequate fathering, Alpha mothering and often parental bullying that quashes self-esteem and creates ego-based relationships. At the risk of being over judg-mental, I will leave this theme for someone who may have more rounded and researched explanations.

Returning to the theme of a black Empathic Approach, there are several compo-nents to consider when addressing black women and self-care. These intersectional components are attached to the impact of racism and internalised racism.

- Be aware of the propensity to assume that Feminist theory fits all women.
- Acknowledge diversity between women in different ethnic groups.
- Notice that racism affects both the subject and perpetrator.
- Complacency. Don't assume that connection with people of colour and black or Asian people means anti-racism.
- Accept that shame or sharam can be a key factor for those impacted by racism.

Shame about skin colour, installed by racism, shame as a woman installed by patriarchy, sexism and misogyny. Shame about powerful unexpressed responses to racism and sexism as an ongoing stigma, linked to the taboo of externalising and challenging racism and other oppressions. Shame connected to skin tone, physical features, hair texture, and dress.

- Drivenness: The ways that she can be task oriented to a point of exhaustion. She continues to take on others' burdens and sometimes not notice when she is experiencing compassion fatigue, or burn out
- Mammying: Taking on the role of teaching and caretaking perpetrators of anti-black racism.
- Compulsive independence: Not asking for help or refusing help when she needs it. Giving the appearance that she can manage on her own.
- Don't discharge messages: Silencing ourselves, not speaking up when she has needs, such as respect for her feelings and support. I have met black women

who pride in appearing stoic and don't allow themselves to be seen crying. She is crying inside.

- Occluded trauma of racism and Sexism.
- Acknowledging that our bodies, our femaleness and sexualities are precious.
- Confronting taboos: Understanding and exploring the multidimensional effect of mistrust, fear, guilt, confusion, ambiguity, shame, self-blame, isolation, internalised anger, internalised sexism & internalised racism, and the silencing nature of oppressions as they impact on self-expression, self-esteem and inter-secting identities of black African/Caribbean/Asian women & families.

Essentially all self-care as black women is key to our ability to experience empathic responses both given and received. What I mean is that if we are not paying full attention to the way we nurture ourselves in a sense of body, mind and spirit, it may be difficult to be fully present, daily with those we are connected to.

Taking time to assess how we are doing with our own caretaking, nurturing, health, boundaries, and demand for respect and loving connections from those in our lives, is a fundamental requirement in our relations with ourselves and others.

It is not always easy to remember that we were born beautiful, and we remain beautiful and tender beneath the harshness of life. Many of us suffer from dys-morphia and low self-esteem due to ways that capitalist, racialised, patriarchal society has influenced attitudes to our body shapes, skin tone and physical features, to name but a few.

We are often marginalised and undermined and internalise these behaviours by not reinforcing our self-care. This discourse engenders grief, sadness and rage, that can lead us into disassociation and often numbness and lack of attention to our self-care. Developing ongoing awareness of our need to be recognised as powerful, yet vulnerable humans, is key to our self-care.

Cooper (2019. P152) believes that rage is a place where black women should begin their healing.

> Black women have the right to be angry. We have been dreaming of freedom and carving out spaces for liberation since we arrived on these shores. We under-stand what it means to love ourselves in a world that hates us, and we know what it means to do a lot with very little.

She quotes 'sass, as in finger waving, eye rolling, attracting laughter'. And she notes that Tyler Perry's Madia and mammy character is a way of expressing anger. She suggests that these are ways that put white people at ease.

Mammying is one of the 'black Western Archetypes', mentioned in book one (Mckenzie-Mavinga 2009). I have always emphasised the importance of BPOC women relinquishing the urge to take care of white people who demonstrate their fragility and hook their peers into a teaching role. Self-care means not being the unpaid tutor, or 'maid' in situations of learning about white people's anti-black racism. Self-care means stepping out of this potential role and harnessing our power, to reinforce energy that affirms our personal and collective well-being. Some BPOC women may not be fully aware of the consequences of slipping into this subservient role. It can be draining and reinforce internalised racism and disempowerment. A black Empathic Approach can support awareness of this, often patterned response, and present an appropriate gaze to assist empowerment and confidence, to say no to these patterns and yes to her self-care.

Cooper (2019. P35) encourages the view that 'black feminism is not about focusing on white damage, it is about a world that black girls can build'.

> 'Black women's rage is a kind of orchestrated fury we've had to learn to move through and use for strength and force and insight within our daily lives. Those of us who did not learn this difficult lesson did not survive. And part of my anger is always libation for my fallen sisters'.
>
> (Cooper 2019. P152)

'However, we know and embrace joy because we know the difference between joy and grief' (PP164–165).

Transforming grief into joy and compassion

April 2023 Tobago

It's Easter Sunday, Ramadan and not yet Passover. I'm in a car with four other local women and one young man. Caroline is driving us to the rainforest. I trust her as she has been my well-being coach for a few years. On a monthly basis, she watches over my vitals and supports me to take care of my body, mind and spirit. I get a full body, well-being session that includes Physical detox, therapeutic massage and cupping. My session with Caroline is usually rounded up with a cup of tea made with either Soursop, Moringa, or Noni leaves.

Today we are heading for main Ridge Tobago, for what Caroline calls rain forest bathing. It's a kind of a meditation while moving through the flora and fauna of the longest protected rainforest in the Western Hemisphere. We drive over the hills taking in the coastline and the vibrant colours of Famboyant and Pui trees. We stop to observe a waterfall, and an ancient silk cotton tree (or Ceiba Pentandra). The Silk Cotton tree is considered sacred as slaves believed their ancestors lived in it. In Asia the tree is called Kapok as its blossom provides insulation, padding in sleeping bags, and stuffing for mattresses and pillows. The tree is magnificent and commanding. If you get close to it, tiny pickers can be seen. I am in awe of this product of Mother Nature towering over us. Her branches spread like wings. She is steadfast. Her roots are unmoved by the wearing elements. The pickers that protrude from her trunk protect the bark that line her inner self. Nature has provided all she needs for her self-care. She provides oxygen and shelter and Ayurvedic healing qualities from her flowers, bark, leaves and roots. I feel protected and have a strong connection. There is similarity in how our own self-care can protect and give us healing, tenderness and strength to connect and assist others to heal.

A discussion ensues, about the closing of a dirt oven, in Castara, a village at the northern end of the Island, that used to serve a variety of local breads and baked products. Caroline thinks out loud about building a dirt oven in her yard. There is plenty of space between the fruit trees, the Noni and Moringa trees and a variety of herbal plants useful for well-being.

When we emerge from the rainforest we share our impressions, while sipping some of Caroline's herbal tea and eating mangoes from her garden. The women I am travelling with are elders like me. We are wise and powerful, and words communicate our Connections. A sense of knowing and support is taken for granted throughout the trip. I feel safe and respected during the few hours we are immersed in nature together, while surrounded by an exhilarating forest blanket. I can breathe. I am in my element. There is no judgement here. It is safe from domineering, controlling oppressions. My glimpse of a benign sense of what it may have been like at birth. Before misogyny, slavery, voluntary servitude, gaslighting got into our systems. Long before the time when I became a victim of compulsive independence and code switching. Long before I realised, I was being treated as a second-class citizen and as though I am made of stone. Long before I worried about eating fat free foods and red meat.

My mind floats back to a previous rainforest trip where we also visited a Hummingbird retreat. My fears about closeness to tiny animals, even insects, were challenged. As we stood in the yard by the feeders, tiny birds of all colours buzzed around me. My body stiffened with terror that I may be landed on or brushed by them. Delight mixed with feelings of resistance consumed me. The retreat manager said that he would show us how to allow the birds to feed from our hands and our heads. My friends stood very still, with arms outstretched and a small feeder had been placed on their hands. The birds came in to feed from them. They flitted away and returned without any harm. Junior placed a feeder on my hand and one on my head. In order to be still I had to relax. I had decided to overcome fears about things, animals, birds that had never harmed me. I breathed deeply and the next thing I knew a Hummingbird had clasped my thumbs with its tiny claws. It drew the sugary fluid from the small pot on my palm and stayed for a few seconds returning repeatedly, for more. This tiny bird felt safe perched on my hand. It trusted me and I trusted myself to be in the moment. At the same time junior had placed a small feeding pot on my head. Although I couldn't see this, a photo was taken as evidence. To others this may seem uncomplicated, but for me it was no mean feat. I was not raised with animals, and I still have mixed feelings about being close with them because they are a different species. I question myself about the similarities of misogyny and racism that separates humans as different species categorised by gender and skin colour. These birds were not biased, they were just hungry and replenishing their energy. There are no words that can really describe my personal growth in this area. I am grateful for Tobago for bringing me closer to nature and to myself. We emerge from the rainforest and share our impressions, while sipping some of Caroline's herbal tea and eating Mangoes from her garden.

Being in nature and being creative have always been essential parts of my self-care and I'm grateful for this connection integrated into my childhood. When I am completely present in nature and there is stillness, I sense a connection with the animals and insects in my environment. This poem was written after one of the rainforest bathing trips.

Rain forest bathing. Main Ridge Tobago (Mckenzie-Mavinga 2022)

I've seen bats cling
between your enclaves
tasted your termites
satiated my guts
with your waters
inebriated,
I breathe, rebirth
peacefully saturated
in silent vigilance
hide and seek clouds
hover.
Stretched limbs
precariously embrace
shadow a soggy crust
beneath rusty leaves
stolen by breeze
strewn carefree
I'm warmed
as sunbeams expose
chequered spaces
silver spinnings
lace over leafy gaps
Tiny beings
tunnel homes
cooperatively ignite
in the underbelly

earth oozes
spring waters
from its umbilicus
baptises cleanse
soothes
I want to
swim naked in you
weave into

your tapestry
To magical cacophony
Parakeets chorus
Chakalaka
announce rain
Mot Mot
perch with poise
only humans
threaten paradise

a benevolent palm
waves
queen-like
In divine connection
taller trees
grandparent saplings
safely spooned
snuggle her trunk
I yearn to share
their cradle

parasitic fingers cling
steeple to heavens
virgin roots twist
tumble-quench-anoint
In this sacred moment

I return home. Back to another reality. A UK news item reported that Diane Abbott had written something about different groups and their experience of racism. There was a huge outcry. A British news channel had reported this issue and they were interviewing white people, mostly men about their views on the hearsay. They were being asked the question, do they think this black woman (who happens to be a long serving MP with a powerful voice) should be suspended? They were not being asked whether they understood the point she was making, but most of them disagreed vehemently with her statement and the hostility was palatable.

Back in the nineties when I was a trainer within predominantly white organisations, many of the participants resisted the idea that white racism exists and is prolific against black people and people of colour. They failed to understand the definition of racism as prejudice plus the power of white privilege, directed systemically, and predominantly towards BPOC individuals. Feminists, those with minority sexualities and those experiencing disablism, claimed a hierarchy of oppressions, that created an initial barrier to accepting the discourses of anti-black, racism. This pain has been minimised, yet it will not go away until perpetrators re-evaluate their responsibilities.

People of any shade of black or brown, and those who ally with anti-racism, fall prey to this insidious oppression. The backlash from media and public influencers seemed vitriolic. A step further than the concern and questioning of Diane Abbot's perspective. There was a huge outcry that seemed to come from lack of acceptance and a hierarchy of oppressions, deeming equal hurt for Jews, Irish, travellers and such like. This confusion is not Diane Abbot's problem, it is a British problem that ripples through the corridors of power, and we get silenced for challenging it.

I felt a gut-wrenching empathy for Diane Abbott, laced with the knowledge that others in power seemed to want to punish her. If a black woman makes a statement in public about the difference between prejudice and racism, they are tarnished. Some of the comments about this apparent political misdemeanour, were thoughtless and in themselves racist and uncompassionate. I heard many assumptions like 'ninety-nine percent of the population would disagree with her comment'.

What gives a white man the authority to speak on my behalf about the difference between racism and prejudice that different groups experience. There was a lot of talk about the past and anti-semitism in the Labour Party. I feared that Diane Abbott's attempts at blaxplaining were taken as anti-Semitic. And I would still like to know which part of it was antisemitic. Was it that she failed to say, 'Jews do experience antisemitism', 'travellers and Irish experience prejudice'. Was it the do, or the don't that crucified her in that moment of committing her thoughts to writing?

The whole incident caused her to quickly apologise rather than clarify the meaning of her statement. It appeared as though she were in a den of lions, and she would be gnarled to death at the slightest vocalisation of her reality. Due to the defensive hierarchy of oppressions, there was no saving her political standing as a black female leader. Even though she attempted to redeem herself the baying hounds wanted to chew her up.

Having not spoken to her personally, but as a black woman in a public leadership role, I feel deeply empathic towards her. This is a black Empathic Approach. I know enough about her as a black woman, to assume the connection between experiencing racism, being silenced, threatened and the possible fear of annihilation.

I wonder what response would have ensued if she had been black and Jewish like me. There was fear in my stomach as I remembered going to a shule with a white Jewish friend and being questioned about my Jewish identity. I noticed my friend was not questioned and I felt humiliated within a community of one part of my heritage. Having to live this experience between two worlds, one African Caribbean, the other black Jewish, has strengthened my resolve that I am one hundred percent of both my heritages. No one can determine that I am half of anything. I have a memory of being surrounded by black girls in secondary school and being questioned about my identity. Am I black or am I half cast? my peers would ask. Looking back, it is clear to see where the questioning has come from and why this had to be a question coming from other minority girls.

This question of identity and colour categories runs throughout my family. My girls who are lighter than me were bullied at school. One of my sons who is darker than me was subject to stereotyping and marginalisation by the schoolteachers and stopped by police under this S.U.S. law at the age of 14. Two of my grandchildren have a white parent and have been subject to racism and shadism during their childhood. Recently one of my daughters called me from her workplace and asked me to help her 'breathe' as she was feeling really traumatised from yet another racist response by a colleague.

Revisiting these experiences has brought me to a point where I feel the need to identify the work I am doing as more than antiracist because I am working with the challenge of white racism specifically because the point of power behind the prejudice of racism can sometimes fix defences and the backlash about this in rigid and unpalatable ways.

I believe that the only way to undermine the power that fixes white racism, whether it be covert or overt, personal or institutional, is to respond with power. So, in a meeting with the challenge of racism workshop facilitators, I spoke about the dangers of white fragility being turned into questioning what racism really is, rather than focusing on the pain and trauma that it causes. Rather than engaging in the process of emerging from the trauma and reclaiming our benign selves as humans. We have been smeared with white racism throughout our lives, and it is time to eliminate racism, anti-Semitism and other forms of oppression. What I am doing here is showing the layers of racism that can occur no matter what status you have in the community. I'm conveying a black Empathic Approach, rooted in my own experience as a black woman. It is on this basis that I encourage the use of this approach to self-care, relational and therapeutic support.

March 2024 Tobago

Today I prepare to visit Caroline for my monthly well-being session. I have always been a physical person and place value on having holistic body work to balance my mental and spiritual state as part of my self-care.

fter a short Reiki meditation, I light candles and oil burners, and I give thanks and ask for blessings at my shrine. Those moments of being fully present, at the start of my day are precious. During that time, I give thanks to the almighty creator for my blessings and achievements. I am grateful for all that contributes to my wellbeing and self-care. My family and friends, my children, my grandchildren and my great grandchildren. I give thanks for my peers, those who accept and overstand alongside the purpose of my work. I give thanks for all the blessings I have received including earth, wind, fire, air, water, minerals and nature and all they contribute to our daily lives. I give thanks for my qualities, my health and fitness, the guardian angels watching over me, my guides and for the ancestors speaking through me with their wisdom, clarity, creativity, congruence, courage and compassion. I do not take these qualities for granted and I do not forget that whatever I am doing in my daily life, there are forces much larger than me.

Caroline always greets me with a hug and a welcoming smile. Becoming aware that I had felt unwell earlier in the week, she offers me a cup of Noni tea. She takes my vitals and checks in with me about how I am and how my life is going and what could have caused my stomach upsets. The upset happened after recognising my compassion overload, after watching the rally to support Diane Abbott, on the news. That day I took out a blank canvas and trickled paint over it as though exorcising my tears. The painting began with a red heart at the centre and then colours took over and tears trickled across the screen. There was a lot of red and blue merged as though the heart had burst and the tears, mostly in white, gave meaning to the shared grief of anti-black racism. (See image on book cover)After the splurge, I felt released.

I became aware of my blood pressure, my heart rate, my weight and how my body was behaving at that moment. We gave time to any imbalance that may have been caused by stress in my life. Then I sank into a bathtub prepared with herbs and essences to detoxify my body. After 25 minutes I am on the couch, giving attention to my lumps and bumps and sore spots. In the background a recording of rain and relaxing music soothes my consciousness. Caroline gives attention to my breathing, while massaging and cupping my sore spots. My mind and body surrender to the healing touch. I drift in and out of consciousness. My trust is renewing. I must be floating somewhere close to when I was born and my benign self allowed sacred holding when I was safe for a short period in my life. Caroline instructs me to do some deep breathing. Then we sat, while drinking some reviving Moringa tea. I leave her home with a renewed sense of well-being and balance of body, mind and spirit, ready to start the day and start over with the purpose of my existence. I have experienced physical, emotional, and spiritual empathy from another black woman, who knows and cares. My trust in humans is reinforced and I am feeling self-compassion.

After meetings with Caroline, I feel at one with myself. Once I arrive home, I take space to allow my self-care to permeate the day and reflect on my surroundings, and my continuing need for nurturing and creative space. The hedges are greener, the sky is a brighter shade of blue. The sounds of the birds and insects have magnified, as though quadraphonic. The air is like a warm blanket. I can slowly return to my daily tasks, including my writing and communication with the outside world. Building compassion is like sipping a glass of warm honey and milk. To savour it and allow it to nourish takes time and attention and most of all conditioning myself to be present in the moment. I think about how I am feeling and ways to maintain calmness and congruence in my day. Once I am interacting with the world my boundaries need to be reinforced. Whilst I am chipping away at the harshness of life, I become more aware of reinforcing joy and tenderness.

March 2024 Tobago

It is Easter Monday, and the latter part of the weekend was spent with a friend on a beach at a local regatta. Another part of the weekend turned out to be rocky, having challenged someone in my personal life, whilst trying to maintain boundaries. I experienced the altercation as misogyny and elder abuse, as the perpetrator happened to be a black male and decades younger than me. I find it helpful to place the type of oppression being experienced, in context.

In response to drawing the line under his unreasonable demands, I received a barrage of disrespect and misogyny. My ongoing self-care and developing capacity to ask for help from close friends, enabled me to remember who I am, and how to take care of myself, in addition to trusting their compassion towards me. I am reminded that my black female friends have got my back, and I reclaim my dignity and courage, and reinforce my right to say NO. When close family members or friends make unreasonable demands or put pressure on me to accommodate their distresses, without offering consideration of my needs and rational discussion. I need help to remember that I am OK as I am, and in my self-care. Noticing where I am receiving compassion from others is key to building my own capacity for compassion. These disruptive interactions enable me to start over and reinforce my selfcare and ability to be compassionate. It is not easy to remember this when we are being disrespected and silenced.

As a theme for the research that I undertook during my MA at Goldsmiths University of London, I decided to use my passion for poetry. As a writer and poet, it had seemed pertinent to explore whether black women were writing about racism and colonialism in their poetry. I discovered early experiences of 'freedom in recalling', expressed in the poetry of a young female slave, Phyllis Wheatly. Wheatly's Poetry is a prime example of creativity and compassion, for herself and collectively. It became a 'symbol of resistance and survival and a voice for millions destroyed in the middle passage'. (London review of books January 2024)

> (Wheatly 1773) 'I, young in life by seeming cruel fate
> was snatched from Afric's fancy'd happy seat
> she goes on to associate mutual liberation from pain
> 'such, such my case.
> And can I then but pray'
> others may never feel tyrannic sway?
> This was an example of reaching out to peers, sharing and breaking the silence
>   and isolation and using writing as a form of self-care.

In the late nineties, I had been teaching students on a PGDIP course in counselling. In some ways I felt that I was an impostor, because I had been invited to teach based on the autobiography that I had published with my sister, about searching for my father's heritage. Perkins & Mckenzie-Mavinga (1991). My name had been dropped by a colleague and my experience of teaching integrative counselling was limited. The course leader said to me, 'just talk about your book'. That was when I realised the connection between breaking out of silence and sharing life stories as a means of connection, counselling and self-care.

Breaking out of the silence that often keeps us shut down and disconnected from others means that barriers of shame or sharam can be shifted. I believe it is important to recognise how shame can incarcerate our minds and bodies. A friend once spoke about his pride, which kept him silent and unable to share his personal pain and hurt. I challenged him to consider the possible difference between 'pride' and the choice to shut down and 'shame' connected to fear and internalised shaming and hurt in our life stories. I realised he was ignoring the shame that he had been harbouring, and he was convincing himself that it was pride that kept him silenced, and limited ways that he could share who he really was.

A black Empathic Approach acknowledges that BPOC individuals have all been shamed in a variety of ways about our skin colour, installed by anti-black racism, and the gendered experiences we share. The shame we harbour as black people and people of colour intersects with shame as women installed by patriarchy, sexism and misogyny. This powerful unexpressed intersection creates ongoing stigma that can crush our self-esteem. Often, we believe this is our normal way of being and internalise hopelessness about being bolder, more open about our life stories and normalising our joy, beauty and courage. Remaining small and emotionally invisible does not serve us, it reinforces stereotypes of worthlessness. The larger picture of who we are can be held by a therapist or supporter who has a firm belief that we are greater than our shame and that we have the potential to transform these negative ways of being, reinforced by internalised racism.

Compulsive independence is another coping pattern, often delivered unconsciously. When we recognise that we are tirelessly worrying about others, yet when it may be appropriate to allow someone to take care of us, some of us behave as though we do not need care and support. It's not difficult to ask for support and say yes when it is being offered. I, for one, have learned that although a little late, as the ageing process kicks in, the real meaning of two heads is better than one and many people make light work.

I used the term 'compulsive independence', because I realise that refusing help can become a debilitating habit that can reinforce isolation and silence. There is no harm in giving ourselves permission to trust others to be involved in what we are doing and create community around us. There is an old saying that no man is an island. When we struggled to voice our needs, when we needed help to walk and talk, and when we needed to learn more, enhance our wisdom, and connect with others for the sake of love, family, and sharing, we trusted ourselves and others to become more informed and connected.

A mixture of oppressions experienced through life created danger signs that challenged our capacity to trust. An epiphany about my mother's abandonment gave me a new insight, that oppression had separated us. This turning point has helped me to reason with the context of how and why humans hurt each other, and we get separated and silenced. This often creates separateness in relationships, sometimes forever. Developing this understanding has given me opportunities to reconnect and trust a renewal of some broken relationships. This has also helped me in my relationships and ruptures with clients.

Silencing ourselves, and not speaking up when we have needs, such as respect for our feelings and support, is a crucial element in holding back on self-care.

I have met black women who don't allow themselves to cry. I cried a lot in my childhood; this became an automatic release for my pent-up feelings. There were times when I cried in silence and times when I bawled out loud. I recognise this form of discharging feelings as a method of self-care, a release from pent-up feelings and cleansing a space for clearer thinking and transformation.

April 2024

Yesterday I travelled to the Island of Saint Vincent. The plan was to spend time there with my youngest son, who is rapidly moving towards his thirty-fifth birthday. When I'm travelling alone, I carry a cane to assist me with balance and inform others that I may walk slowly and be less able in some situations. I am less conscious of being gawked at and questioned and more aware that help is available if needed. The airlines are improving on their ability to accommodate most forms of disability. Some of the young men address me as 'mummy'. It feels respectful and endearing. It connects me to the village, and I feel respected as their elder.

My son has requested that I support him to connect with a missing part of his childhood. We often visited his father's land when he was a child. This time he is a man choosing to bear his grief by honouring his father's place of rest. Having not had this opportunity with my own father, I have high respect for his decision. As his mother, I am proud to acknowledge his ability to ask for support as a young man, taking charge of his life, his heritage and future. He comes across as a quiet person and I notice he seems contained and uses his integrity when he needs to challenge a situation. I wonder if he has inherited that reserved part of me that others have noticed. I am also aware we both catch on to deep meaning and usually respond openly. He has a good sense of humour. I am not sure about this trait in myself, because I don't often get jokes. I celebrate our diversity and learn from it. Having sent him to learn about rites of passage at the age of thirteen, with a group of black men, I value the way he is able to challenge me and speak his truth. I learned not to interrogate him or intrude on his privacy and wisdom as a young man. I remember him requesting that I no longer choose his clothes or his books. This was an enlightenment about subtle ways of emasculation. He would no longer allow me to conquer his imagination. He learned how to separate from and challenge his mother respectfully and this enabled me to more easily accept the distance that grew between us as he matured into a young man.

I have learned about my own self-care as a priority in parenting and perpetrating equality within my family, especially with my sons and grandsons. This was another level of awareness towards men in general. I became super aware of the mistakes I had made in relationships with the men in my life. I am also starkly aware of the repair work I needed to do, and the levels of radical self-care needed for my recovery. Speaking up about self-care and love should be equal, so that we can balance and feel confident in the ways we present to others.

I notice how women are available to support each other when things go wrong and, in my experience, we rarely challenge each other about our attitudes towards men. Is this another form of silence and internalised sexism? Having to check myself in this area means spending time on the process or sharing my compassion with men and working through where it gets difficult. This process means remembering that I was innocent when I became a victim of misogyny, sexism and racism and being compassionate about my injuries from oppressive experiences. Thus, being compassionate towards myself to the best of my ability means I can achieve a level of compassion towards others. Readers may see how huge this topic is, so I am chipping away at it and sharing how my personal experience is an important element contributing to a black Empathic Approach.

The use of a three-dimensional approach may be necessary in portraying this context of empathy. Whilst intuition may connect the subject of racism with the therapist, an objective stance that draws on knowledge of the systemic and traumatic nature of anti-black racism can support a holistic and connecting aspect of this beast. The third dimension of this approach draws on the therapist's ability to dialogue confidently about their knowledge and overstanding of how racism infiltrates the subject's confidence and ability to manage their coping responses to any form of oppression. It is important to hold and account for feelings, responses and coping modes evoked by racism. Thinking about empathy in diverse integrative ways is useful when applying a black empathic approach.

> Objective empathy involves going beyond merely calculating and evaluating items from a self-report personality inventory or completing a rote scanning of a behavioural checklist in order to categorise the psychopathology of a client. Instead, a practitioner assumes an empathic position of objectively derived findings to illuminate what life is like for an individual in lived contexts.
>
> Clarke (2022. P35)

Considering that the focus on a black Empathic Approach is concerned with the impact of anti-black racism, it would be viewed as an 'emic' approach, rather than 'etic'. A generalisation that assumes an approach transcending all cultures. This approach encourages a mindset that assists inquiry into how the specific oppression of anti-black racism impacts in personal and systemic ways.

A client became aware of her fear of rejection from her family if she shared with them how racism and shadism within the family silenced her and minimised her experiences as 'the darkest one'. Witnessing the pain of her internalised racism, I assured her that I was watching her back, during her process of making a decision to find her own voice, so that she could address the growing distance between herself and her siblings. I used intuition and a compassionate stance to let her know that I suspected she was feeling hurt about the nature of her relationships within the family and how this impacted her as a black woman.

My personal knowledge and experience of anti-black racism and internalised racism was useful for an objective stance. This helped her engage in a context for discussion and further enquiry about her situation. She then became aware that the situation is common and known to evoke isolation. During further meetings, we were able to consider ways that she can be less isolated and forge future support to externalise her thoughts and feelings in safe spaces, where there is likely to be acceptance rather than denial of the reality and commonality of racism and internalised racism. A compassionate stance is needed to deeply connect with this kind of experience and show the subject of racism robust holding and support.

Summary

Self-care is essential to the process of minimising the gap between rage and compassion. The first step is accepting the importance of moving along this spectrum in order to bring about creative boundaries in our thinking and behaviour. The journey to achieving this requires a determination to break old habits of cooperating with ways that racism can maim ways of being. The courage to take this in hand, and know and create confidence in ourselves, means taking steps to break colonial boundaries that can create binary thinking in the ways we approach meaningful therapeutic and supportive relationships where racism is present. BPOC women have many models of radical self-care that encourage their ways of being. I found Lorde's book, 'The uses of anger', Coopers book, 'Eloquent Rage', and my former literature mentors, Angela Davis, Maya Angelou, bell Hooks, and many more encouraging writers, assisted me along the way. I feel encouraged that as I complete this chapter, The US hada black female candidate running for presidential election. We now have a female president and Prime Minister in Trinidad and Tobago, and Barbados President Mia Mottley to name but a few encouraging role models, in our midst.

This chapter is dedicated to BPOC Pioneers of Mental and Physical Health. Baroness Ros Howells, Mavis Best, Sybil Phoenix, Diane Abbot, and others who paved the way in London and the UK.

Chapter 11

A work in progress

Workshops on a black Empathic Approach are in demand. I am grateful to the Black African and Asian Therapy Network, its leadership group, and the membership who have noticed and supported the development of my work from its inception. Eugene and Jayakara Ellis were especially helpful when my books were taking root.

Makemba Kunle, a renowned Trinidadian artist and friend, offered his Art centre in Trinidad for the launch of my second book. 'The Challenge of Racism in Therapeutic Practice' (2016). Local creatives in the Art world and leaders such as Leroy Clarke attended. They showed appreciation which had not been forthcoming in my place of work, where I was teaching, in the UK and where the bulk of the research took place. I was refused sabbatical and my writing was not celebrated; However, I was honoured in the land of my late father and felt as though I had a place in my ancestral home. This part of my journey helped to fill a missing link in my heritage, that I discovered and claimed with my sister in 1984. Mckenzie-Mavinga and Perkins (1991) This was a completeness that soothed my grief and cradled my rage.

There are no words to explain the discovery of my Father's Trinidadian family. They welcomed me unconditionally and I have since experienced a deep loving connection with them. I learned about compassionate family acceptance, in all our diversity. My late Trinidadian sister, and her East Indian husband, showed me the meaning of family love, that continues through the love and acceptance shared by their remaining nine children and extended family. I cannot explain the joy and fulfilment in my heart when I am cradled within this huge family of four generations.

Through my writing I embraced a new part of my development, that of allowing the community to support me, led by individuals who appreciated my work. Empathy was shown to me as I navigated the neglect of the education system that I thought I belonged to. I realise it was the students that really appreciated my contribution. I was fortunate that they allowed me to engage with them in the systemic neglect of their learning needs, in terms of the effects of anti-black racism. The staff were relieved, because I was filling a gap that showed their inadequacies. I had been quietly burrowing a channel for opening this dialogue.

DOI: 10.4324/9781003479994-12

My rage was kept under wraps, whilst cautiously I engaged with those likely to be on the front line of the mental health system. Before I was given the opportunity to teach, I worked at the African Caribbean Mental Health Association in Brixton, South London. The befriending work founded by Errol Francis in the 80s and 90s was taking root. The association offered individuals captured by the mental health system a black Empathic Approach to their care, by nature of an 'appropriate gaze'. Clients said it felt like 'home from home', as they encountered care and support offered by people who looked like them and could reflect a gaze that demonstrated connection and knowledge about systemic racism.

It turned out that the management were treated like puppets by the local authority, to pacify the systemic racism in mental health care. Demands from staff for support, recognition and resources were being ignored. Accountability for the ongoing development and budget for the project failed and as a group, we challenged the management. Subsequently, I became one of five staff who were suspended without notice or pay. It was messy, unethical and wounding. The project had imploded. After several court appearances we were offered compensation. I never received a penny of the £9000 compensation awarded to me. I felt exploited and enraged, particularly because these were my own people. With support, I let it go and moved on.

One door closed and the door of teaching opened. I started teaching at Southwark College, followed by City University and Goldsmiths University of London. This led me to a senior lecturer position at London Metropolitan University. I felt marginalised within the staff team and tokenised as the only person of colour in the department.

In addition to teaching, I offered counselling to a variety of students, many of them were international students who had fled their homelands in terror and were seeking refuge. I knew that my contribution was influential, and at that early stage in my career, my rage began to turn to compassion. I believe this transformation was spurred by the recognition of what I had to offer as a black woman.

Tobago May 2024

It's 3:00 AM on a Sunday morning. Having retired early, I am awake. The book is on my mind. I'm working through the first draft and keen to move on, but I don't know what to say. I thought I had retired, yet there is a demand to carry on and see this through. I started this book with the intention of creating a legacy that would influence the field of psychotherapy and counselling. There are many influencers who have joined this discourse, and I no longer feel alone. We are singing the same song with different yet similar words. Some call it anti-colonialism. Some still call it multiculturalism and blend intersectional contexts. I stand firmly by the cause of anti-racism, until this cruel figment of our past wears itself out. My journey from rage to compassion is incomplete. It is ongoing and I am living through the experience. There is still much silence, and I continue to speak and express the need to specifically address the impact of anti-black racism. How else can this blight be healed?

The rage within me is quieter but not dampened. It flickers like an ember that can be reignited at any point. Tempered by my growing compassion, I am aware that balance can be created by accepting the normality of rage and knowing that compassion can be revised and relearned for it to be allowed and given its place. There is a place for compassion to grow amongst the weeds of racism, that tangle and choke the sensitivity of human life.

Living the cause of a black Empathic Approach and bearing witness to the growth and development of others working with this process helps to feed this concept into the world. Most of the time spent writing this book I have been away from the UK, the place of its inception. I have created distance that gave me an opportunity to bathe my mental well-being in the elements and look across thousands of miles to where I have lived the rage of a black woman growing and suffering with the intersectionality of racism. So, what was it all about? My personal journey was isolating, yet encouraged and supported in these latter years, by colleagues and peers and those who have journeyed alongside me and been willing to learn about the concept of a black Empathic Approach.

I discovered literature about rage, when previously I was unaware that anything had been written about it. The first time I read about rage as permissible and justified, was in Pinkola Estes' book (1996), Women Who Run with The Wolves. There was a piece written about 'rage as a teacher'. (P352) 'All emotion, even rage, carries knowledge, insight, what some call enlightenment. Our rage can, for a time, become our teacher, a thing not to be rid of so fast … The cycle of rage is like any other cycle; it rises, falls, dies and is released as new energy'.

I gained permission to learn about how I can accept my rage and make it productive. Those around me noticed my rage, and I am aware that at times it must have appeared ferocious or reminded them of their own rage stuffed down and unattended to. Once I have let off steam, I become fully aware of the hurt lying underneath that grips my throat like barbed wire. My vulnerability manifests and I feel like a small child who needs to be handled delicately. The tears come and only then it seems can others see the whole of me in my fragility. I often wonder, what is it that prevents others noticing the vulnerability of black women?

How long do we harbour our feelings inside before it is safe enough to show them. In the West we harbour compressed shame about really showing ourselves and revealing injuries and taunts from the past. I have encountered these blockages when working with clients. My therapy training did not include working with shame and rage as potent themes. These themes are relevant to lifelong oppressions that individuals experience. Training silenced the existence of internalised racism and the subjects and perpetrators of its demeaning power. I am one who missed out on safe spaces to gain strength from support and education in this area.

I had never really expressed my rage whilst learning to become a therapist. No one knew about the feeling of barbed wire in my throat, but later in a therapy session, I recalled the time when a man tried to strangle me. This was a realisation of my traumatic intersection of misogyny and anti-black racism.

Rage has now become my teacher, and I have learned that this powerful feeling is a normal response to an abnormal situation. The injustices of racism, misogynoir and heteronormativity are rife. I am still afraid of being rejected and the abandonment that can be projected towards me when I show my rage. I continue to be aware that I can also project rage. Sometimes it blurts out and before I know it, others have noticed. It is attached to stuff from my early years and so much life experience that I have brought along with me. As I continue to chip away at it and the effect that this has on myself and others, I notice that most of all, it is possible to live with the scars of the past and create healing pathways for our existence. One of those pathways is compassion.

My rage about being abandoned soon after entering the world and subsequent emotional neglect was more like righteous indignation. I was entitled to the full family experience that never happened. I raged about the isolation, lack of acknowledgment and being unchosen. My rage at betrayal, lack of acceptance and undermining in my marriage was righteous indignation. The grief and loss of pregnancy termination, after violence in a subsequent relationship was righteous indignation. And that isn't all.

Lorde (2007) (in Alexander & Sheftall), 'The uses of anger' P6,

anger is not a sign of (black women's) weakness of character, nor is it a psychological defect. Instead, it is about entrenched racism, anti-black violence, unjust institutions and the refusal of (white) feminists to engage in an honest conversation about these problems. Anger can be a transformative catalyst for change.

Lorde addressed the repeated messages of being 'unchosen' that black girls and women face, thus resulting in anger and being expected to live an ordinary life or perish. She identifies the silence and collusion of white women's evasion of facing what our rage means.

Perpetrators tend to dilute challenges about their anti-black racism. They turn away from it and deny their privilege as a way of silencing and escape from facing our pain with us. For that reason, I have had difficulty trusting deep lifelong allyship with white people. The business of calling out their racism and collusion without being subject to their privilege and fragility can be tricky in training situations, for BPOC individuals, so this conflict is often avoided. How then can we learn from each other if we are avoiding the crux of the problem? What does it take for us to decide to lean into hard talk about the personal effects of racism and come out the other end better informed?

Lorde goes on to address how internalised racism can get in the way and cause evasion between black women and women of colour. She suggests that (Lorde (2007. P169, in Alexander & Sheftall. P15) 'the road to anger is paved with our unexpressed fear of each other's judgement'. Although the focus of her analysis is black American women, there is little difference in the ways that 'shadism' as one portion of our intrinsic oppressions and diversity is riveted into the existence of BPOC individuals.

I have learned greater trust in my intuition and ways to create stronger boundaries to protect my emotional and physical well-being. Learning from my rage is central to my self-care and integrity. We learn from our position in our families, education systems, workplaces and social situations, that we are categorised by our levels of blackness, hair texture, hierarchy of opportunities associated with femaleness, maleness and biological feminine opportunities. I write from my experience as a black woman and do not apologise for this.

The misogynoir that black women and women of colour face contributes to our self-concept and ability to be powerful with our oppressors and with each other. Lorde (2007. P168) in Alexander & Sheftall (P16). views anger as a way of keeping people separate when connection is already limited. She suggests that

> we must analyse the truth in our levels of self-care, so that our ability to love another black person and see one's own face in their reflection is not tarnished. So that we can offer the same love of ourselves as black women and women of colour, to our sisters and brothers. As our anger diminishes our ability for compassion and love grows.

I want to tell you about where this perspective of a black Empathic Approach was birthed, and how it has been growing over the past 30 years. The concept manifested in my initial research and practice with professionals, trainees, students, supervisees and also clients.

At the time I was challenged by my own training as the only person of colour and my experiences of racism within the training.

My experiences of not feeling I had a voice and not being recognised in terms of my identity, as a black woman, experiencing racism in my life, and on the training. My research kicked off when I was a senior lecturer at one University in London while also visiting two other Universities to support tutors in thinking about changing their attitude but also to assist students to think differently about working with the impact of racism.

The research that I initially carried out for my doctorate, which was recorded in my first book 'Black Issues in the Therapeutic Process' (2009) showed the necessity of addressing racism and black issues. I'm now in the process of working with a hypothesis which advances this discourse that I have found myself immersed in. The hypothesis suggests that if we change the attitude and mindset of educators, particularly those who are working in the field of psychotherapy and relational contexts, we can challenge them to think differently about one of the generic areas of therapeutic and relational support, namely 'empathy'. Then we can create something that is not solely built on introjection or projections connected to fear and powerful feelings about racism. Once this is happening, and this is what I propose in the workshops, I believe that it is possible to work together to heal the collective discourse of racialisation and pain associated with antiblack racism. This has brought us to the concept of a black Empathic Approach.

The concept needed to stand alone and be seen as purposeful when listening and attending to the dilemma of racialisation and systemic racism. It is unique in that my expectation of its use requires a clear understanding that racism becomes internalised. Being unaware or unwilling to address its impact on relational processes can mean collusion or perpetration of the trauma that it can create. This concept demands more than a recognition of oppression.

Realising that racism is installed in systemic DNA, means that Western cultures are saturated in it. We are compelled to live within these systems, and our liberation depends on making decisions about interrupting, challenging and personally eliminating the damage that racism can cause.

There is a difference between 'cultural empathy' and a black Empathic Approach. We cannot take for granted that cultural empathy sufficiently addresses racism. A black Empathic Approach is anti-racist in nature because of its deliberate action to address anti-black racism. This approach draws on therapists' or supporters' capacity and robustness to address anti-black racism contexts and racialised processes.

Doing this work alongside having a life and being part of everyday family life and village struggles meant I had to remove myself from certain elements of life, toxicities, and negatives that influence my well-being. As a vulnerable human being, I am entitled to protect myself from the risk of reintroducing the disease of racism. This is my first line of self-care. When there is no love, when recognition of my joys and struggles is limited, I stay quietly on the sidelines.

I am still enraged. Ongoing support from the Re-evaluation Co-counselling Community, doing yoga and my Reiki practice offer tools that support me. In these circles, I encounter individuals who trust the community to hold and assist them in expelling the distresses and negative patterns that chain them to the past as perpetrators and subjects of racism. The Re-evaluation Co-counselling Community is built on a history of eliminating damage caused by oppressions, and there are pockets within the practice for safety to address specific oppressions, and movement towards liberation.

Reiki is a more meditative spiritual discourse that does not openly address diversity and oppression. In these groups, I am often in a minority as a person of colour, so I am supported in the process of deep relaxation and introspection, which balances and calms me, as does my yoga practice. Friends and peers often refer to my calm demeanour. I have no idea of their projections and what this means to them. Can it be that they misunderstand my stillness? Do they have any idea of the tempered furnace of injustice, inside me?

One of the Reiki principles suggests 'Just for today do not anger'. Although this is an invitation to calm feelings of resentment and rage, I struggle with this principle. If I am angry, I am angry and I do not believe anyone should be instructed not to express this feeling. Of course, in some circumstances, modification in terms of our expression of anger may be needed. However, I see the possibility that expressing rage, rather than becoming depressed is likely to be a healthier option, once support for recovery is available. I believe that after a seething rage humans need soothing contact. Being judgmental about rage does not help to soothe it. We have personal responsibility and choice to learn from rage.

Transforming rage into compassion for myself and others was another stage in my personal development and therapeutic practice. As with empathy, compassion cannot be switched on and off. It is a component that comes from an open heart. It is a genuine reaching out and something we can be, not something we can do. An open heart is part of a journey that allows for vulnerability and deep connection to occur and show itself to others. It is not intellectual or academic, it is human. It lacks pretence and is not the same as sympathy. I have become curious about what others were saying about compassion.

Learning about compassion has been key in this stage of my personal journey. I needed mentoring so I turned to a book written by Desmond Tutu. 'The Book of Forgiving' (2015). This is a courageous story of overcoming the brutality of murder, deception and the pain of grief associated with the tragedies caused by racism and Apartheid in South Africa. Tutu suggests that we have the potential to use pain for healing.

Alleyne (2022. P221) 'There are very few references to compassion in situations when coping with racism. Increased compassion can enable easier access to others suffering and pain, particularly in the mental and psychological health professions when racism is apparent'.

Professor Paul Gilbert (2013. P13) explains how

a process of developing compassion for the self and others increases well-being and aids recovery. Compassion can be defined in many ways, but its essence is a basic kindness, with a deep awareness of the suffering of oneself and of other living things, coupled with the wish and effort to relieve it.

Gilbert (2013. P13)

Developing compassion for oneself and others can help us face up to and win through hardship and find a sense of inner peace. However, in modern societies, we rarely focus on this key process that underpins successful coping and happiness and we can be quick to dismiss the impact of modern living on our minds and well-being. Instead, we concentrate on doing, achieving and having'. Our minds have developed to be highly sensitive and quick to react to perceived threats and this fast-acting threat-response system can be a source of anxiety, depression and aggression. Not only does compassion help to soothe distressing emotions, but it also actually increases feelings of contentment and well-being.

Gilbert (2013. P28)

Being compassionate is not a soft option or just 'being nice'. It can be very difficult, because it means standing up to some of our own desires and refusing to act on some of our lusts or fears. It can also mean recognising that an intense desire for belonging and connectedness to be one of a tribe and defend our own interests, can be the source of intense cruelty and atrocity. The tough issue in compassionate behaviour is addressing our own inner tendency towards cruelty.

I needed to own up to my need for revenge towards those unable to accept the lived experience of anti-black racism and its systemic perpetration. My angry feelings toward those who silence themselves, or remain bystanders, watchers and collude with racism do not serve me and cannot support a black Empathic Approach. I had to find ways of being forgiving, more accepting and engaging my own learning. Each racist encounter demands greater self-care and self-compassion.

The connection between compassion and self-care is important. Self-compassion can enable us to move away from self-criticism. To greater self-esteem. The effect of guilt can be burdensome and create unhealthy behaviours of wanting to pacify others by being in servitude. These attitudes can lead to envy of others because of feeling bad about ourselves. These feelings do not work as a temporary fix. They do not create barriers to protect us against feelings of inadequacy and dissatisfaction with our lives. Imposter syndrome is one such mode of undermining confidence, when we do not feel up to a task that we are performing, yet often we are unable to figure out what may have caused this inadequacy.

Harnessing self-compassion and recognising our power can help. Developing compassion is different from developing a compassionate mind. This is because compassion is more than just thinking. 'I understand, or I know what you are going through'. To behave in compassionate ways, we need to turn off the angry or sad brain and allow a warm heart that genuinely connects. There is no magic switch to turn it on and off. It consists of self-knowledge, self-care, self-love and warmth.

Tutu and Tutu (2015) explain how revenge, vindictiveness, harbouring hurt, resentment and causing self-injury do not serve us, or anyone else. I believe that these emotions are the basis of hatred. It has been suggested that these actions are like 'throwing daggers at someone whilst killing ourselves'. Whilst I get this statement, I am not even halfway towards turning my hurt into profitable self-care.

On two different occasions this week I experienced vitriolic behaviour towards me whilst I was feeling that I was the innocent party. Gaslighting and hurtful attitudes made me feel abandoned and disrespected on a deep level. I was being dumped on. My instinct was to run for cover. In both circumstances I attempted to reason with the other person and request a respectable loving discussion. That was not going to happen, because the other party was determined that I was in the wrong, not that I had made a mistake, or could redeem myself if I had been fully aware of how being me had caused their upset. This is where continuing to communicate in a respectful non defensive way offers the possibility of change in the relational process.

Compassion was out of our reach, and I felt enraged at the loss of love in what I believed was friendship. In one of those relationships, I feel that the friendship is damaged beyond repair, because I was not given a chance to know and understand my part in the conflict. I experienced silence and being silenced and felt kicked to the curb. In the other relationship we are bound by family ties, and I have decided to be patient until the relationship can heal. I have experience of this working in the past. Time can be a healer. These ruptures can be painful and require self-care and self-love to heal the wounds and rebuild confidence. Once I asked a man what is the best way to resolve conflict with men? He answered, 'Keep talking'. Of course, I accept that this is not always possible, if the other party refuses to talk. Therefore, the relationship is blocked.

Although these were personal relationships, I carry the hope of lovingly resolving conflict into my training work. I am aware that fundamentally we are all good human beings. We just get saturated with hurt and oppression, that causes us to hurt others, including those we love. It's not easy to hold on to this belief, when you are a subject of oppressions and systemic racism, but I believe it is possible. Being non-judgmental and facing the challenges together, means we are supported and in agreement, in the process of eliminating the trauma of racism. Compassion is a resource in our emotional tool bag, and we can choose to draw on it when necessary. I believe that if we practise this strategy, shifts in dialogue and relationships influenced by the impact of racism can be affected.

My developing relationships with animals, insects and tiny beings has given me keys to how far I have come and how far I need to travel on the road to compassion. Unlocking this process is challenging. These are the keys to the heart of my emotional responses, to something very different in size, shape and colour. These are the keys to unlocking prejudice and fears and maybe my terror of the dark. I am aware this may take a lifetime.

2022 UK

During my first equine experience, in a field in Bedfordshire, four Pregnant mares had been invited to share the human experience. I came face to face with my childhood isolation and vulnerability. Many years ago, I rode a horse in a group and fed a horse an apple over a fence in a field. Now I was being invited into the field, to make closer contact. The horses seemed friendly whilst left alone on the other side of the fence. This was not long after I'd had knee surgery. There were three tutors supporting the group. Although we were told that it was a team effort, I felt alone. There were two members of the group who were more experienced than me.

I was encouraged by D, the only black female Equine therapist that I know of. She modelled closeness by calmly reaching her hands out and making close physical contact with some of the horses. Her partner squatted down and allowed a horse to investigate his hat. I felt terrified seeing a horse towering over him. I considered him to be brave and fearless.

It took me a while to enter the field, as I noticed that there were more horses in the field than people. One of the tutors assured me I could take my time to go inside. She had given me a plastic box that I could take with me, if I felt like doing so. I felt they were watching my back from a few yards away. Tentatively, carrying the box,

I went inside the field. A couple of horses came across to greet me. I patted them gingerly and noticed there was eye contact. I had put the box down beside me. One of the horses moved towards the box and pounded a hoof on it, pushing it towards me. I understood this to mean that I could sit if I wanted. I was afraid and I did not want the horse to be towering over me. A tutor explained that this horse had been raising her left back leg, in sync with my left knee injury. I experienced this gesture as empathy and an incredible connection.

There was a point in the experience where I sat inside an enclosure and observed the situation and reflected on myself. It was cathartic and the tears flowed.

A tutor suggested that the horse with a mixed brown and white mane, that stayed separate from the group, represented me. I recognised this as an interpretation of the way I often stay separate, noticing my difference, as a mixed heritage brown skinned woman, and the significance of being raised away from my family. In many ways, that day was an epiphany. I got close to animals much bigger than me. They offered me contact. I allowed them closeness to a point where they offered empathic responses. There was diversity and compassion in the responses. I learned about my terror of otherness, and how I make myself small and powerless as a coping skill, when I am afraid of something that appears much bigger than me. I saw clearly how my past had affected my present. I released, pent up tears and feelings of isolation. I took another step to show my vulnerability and allow others to support and encourage me.

My second equine experience took place in a larger, more diverse group. I was determined to be bolder and less afraid of closeness with the big animals. It was another moving experience that showed me the horses were rivalling for my attention and wanted to get close and be playful. I was open to learning more about the horses and myself. This experience was more empowering in that I had decided to build on what I had learned in the first meeting. Once again It was humbling and reflected my feelings of isolation in a group. I was able to get close to more than one horse at the same time, without feeling terrified. They were attentive and patient. I spoke more and affirmed the horses. Perhaps a step to becoming more engaged. I was not previously aware of how paralysing fear can be and of my own fear in taking another step.

2023 Tobago

In thinking about tiny animals and insects. I had an experience last year where I agreed to let some hummingbirds feed from my hands and perch on my head. There were others in the group who seemed fearless about doing this, but it took me a while to pluck up the courage and become less afraid of the speed and whirring of their wings, as they fluttered in and out of my space. It took patience and courage not to be alarmed when a bird perched on my hand and grabbed my thumb with its claws. I noticed its confidence and security, as perching on my hand gave the bird security to feed. I stilled my hand and body and allowed this moment of mutual security. I needed to trust being still and just allow them to be momentarily close to me. Past trauma manifests in many ways. These sacred moments of stillness and mutual healing have become precious. I am beginning to unpick my hypervigilance and discover the meaning of meditation.

On another occasion, a little girl held out a box with tiny chicks in it. She came towards me and asked me if I wanted to hold one. She knew nothing about my fears and past traumas. Not noticing my fear, she took a chick out-of-the-box and put it in my hand. I had little chance to refuse her wish. It seemed that she trusted her own relationship with tiny animals and in her innocence, she had not expected me to be afraid of holding this small being. I learned that she had trust in me and trust in the small vulnerable birds. I could have screamed, or dropped it, But I stayed with the experience and allowed my stillness and compassion to overcome my embarrassment and resistance as an adult.

Having witnessed other adults being gentle with insects I am more aware of how my response to them is conditioned by fear. Although insects can be invasive and sometimes hurt humans in their quest for survival, I am practising ways to be less harsh in my response to them. They have a purpose and share the land with us, and we as larger beings can be cruel in our attempts to clear them from our human space.

There is a Reiki principle that challenges my relationship with animals and insects. 'Show gratitude to every living thing'. This is a huge challenge for me, as I do not feel equal to animals and insects. I often feel fear and disgust. On reflection, there is little difference between my attitude and attitudes that generate hate crimes, the violence of war, genocide and ethnic cleansing? I am learning that compassion already existed within me. I just needed to harness it. I am a work in progress.

Chapter 12

The legacy, a black Empathic Approach

In considering key elements of accepting the oppression that white privilege and white fragility can cause, there is no argument that compassion, congruence, courage and knowledge of oneself and one's ability to dialogue about this oppression in non-defensive ways, is important to a black Empathic Approach. To therapists who ask how do you do this? I say to you, learn about your own ethnicity, your own skin colour and your own hurts with regards to anti-black racism, and develop a robust approach to working with this concept in personal development and well-being. This book arose from a wish to create a legacy of my work in promoting and modelling a black Empathic Approach.

I am still wondering how I arrived at the point of achieving this part of my heritage. I believe it shows what is possible and documents what may seem impossible, because of the emotional load that runs alongside the story of developing a black Empathic Approach.

In some ways, it has been a journey of blood, sweat and tears. Revealing parts of my story, and our history has meant that I have been reliving poignant areas of growth, from rage to compassion. My rage has been too silent for too long and as it has become manifest through my writing, the risks of exposure and fear of personal annihilation have become more real.

Like Anne, many tangible influences of my work have shown up spontaneously during this process. I will present the final part of our dialogue to demonstrate this.

Concluding Anne's interview with me

Dr. Isha: People would come up to me and say, 'you saved my life' and I'm thinking what do you mean? you saved your own life. It was Just a few words, and it became natural after that. If it works once, it will always work. It's just about connection and seeing the other human being. I cannot say that I'm never angry with my people, because I do get angry, I cannot say that I never want to be in spaces that are predominantly white. I'm seventy-five and I'm beginning to feel confident about being the only one because I am still in some of these spaces and knowing I'm spiritually protected.

DOI: 10.4324/9781003479994-13

It feels like you are an Angel, because as a white person, you are giving me an appropriate gaze which is rare. It takes risk and it takes courage, and I pray for courage every day in the work that I'm doing. It takes courage to take it and run with it.

Anne: I'm going to pause because I feel very moved by hearing you say that, and this time I am able to receive it without having to wait weeks. The bravery, I've known you for a while and you know I've gotten to know you much better after our supervision, and I haven't heard you tell your story quite like that. What has continued to come up for me as you've been speaking, is how brave you must have been for your whole life. When you said I'm still summoning this bravery and praying for bravery, I was thinking well if you're still trying to get it, who's got it? I'm also wondering what it's like to retire and what it's like to start putting some of this work down. Also, what it's like for part of your retirement to be in a place where you are not the only black person.

Dr. Isha: Important questions you can hear my voice softening as I begin to consider your questions about retirement, because I've retired from one to one and group psychotherapy and supervision. I consider myself retired from the battle but what brought me through this is the use of my voice. I don't believe I'm a massive campaigner, but I work on this through my writing. The two preceding books and bringing forward what I call a black Empathic Approach, this is my life story. This is how I got to this point. Compassion is key to a black Empathic Approach, and you have started noticing that for yourself. I believe that compassion is something we can all achieve, but sometimes life stories get in the way of feeling it for ourselves and showing it to others. I am still a work in progress. I thought I had retired completely. I wanted to stop writing anything academic. I wanted to stop doing any teaching or sharing or showing people how to do this, but I set it up so that it's not like that.

A Nigerian man said to me, when I told him that I am going to retire, that 'when you publish a book you are responsible for the readers and I said "no no no no no, I'm retiring". But I realise it's absolutely true, so I'm working on legacy now and I'm saying hopefully this is a final book, about developing the black Empathic Approach, which is key to what we are talking about. That's what it is in one sentence. It's a black Empathic Approach. I'm considering that as my legacy.

I'm also supporting the Master Facilitators that I have trained in doing the Challenge of Racism workshops, to assist therapists to integrate concepts that were brought forward in the books, and to learn how to do this. To learn to find the compassion to do this. That's my legacy and some of them are becoming robust in teaching this and I'm happy that the work is going to go forward in this way. It's already going forward in this way and people can teach what I felt was needed for this work and bring it forward and keep transforming the field.

Anne: What's it like to retire somewhere where you're not the only black person so first of all tell us where you are with all this sunshine that's streaming in behind you, and the birds chirping in the background, because it's not England.

I'm on the sunny Paradise Island of Tobago. I'm here in my ancestral home for part of my year and I am still writing. I want to find the time to publish a poetry collection. I've always written poetry from a young age and that has helped me through a lot of self-expression. I'm away here, but I am deep into the international process of living in the village so to speak. The village of predominantly black African heritage peoples.

The Trinidad and Tobago population boasts a mixture of Indian and African peoples, a proportion of mixed peoples and Chinese people. Tobago is populated by many families of black African heritage. I see very clearly how the internalised racism and colonialism has injured many people here because it comes out in how they hurt each other, and how they behave to each other across and within the cultural divides. It is also very apparent in how they protect each other, and how the village is like one family. I'm living here. This is a bonus. People watch me. I know that they're watching to see if I'm ok. The Roosters are watching too. I can hear them, like they come here in my yard. Like a family, they have high expectations that I will feed them.

Anne: I have two last questions. My first one is you said this book and this work is your legacy. What is it like to have a very tangible legacy to leave behind, meaning there are already people like me. A lot of the therapists that I work with speak about you in hushed tones. Your book is available on most bookstore shelves, and you've changed the way that people work. You've changed this industry without question, and what is that like for you?

Dr. Isha: I feel there's still a lot of work to be done, because people are doing it. I also think there's still a lot of insecurity because of institutions. Some of them are transforming and have taken it on board but not enough money is being put into supporting the learning system to just do it. There are too many excuses as to why it can't be done now. That's very evident in the number of organisations that want the training. They want to learn this, but they don't want to pay for it. They have these financial restrictions. They don't want to buy something that's going to be transformative for their organisations and for the senior people working in their organisations, so that they can pass it on to the next generations. It's too slow but it's trickling in if this is how it must happen, and there's some people who are determined to take it forward, it may happen eventually. Many people know I'm not the only one that's doing this work but the way in which I'm doing it is different and profound. What was the question again? How it feels to be leaving behind a tangible legacy. I feel pleased about that. I'm committed to seeing this through so that it's here when I'm not here, but it carries on. I'm not Freud but I don't mind if people call my name like they called Freud's name.

Anne: You're less problematic than Sigmund Freud, so we do well to replace him. It already happens. I hear your name get dropped a lot and in my head I'm always like, thinking, that's my supervisor you know. Some people have probably grown quite weary of hearing me brag about it, but I'm always very proud to say that I worked with you, so thank you.

Dr. Isha: You will pop the legacy the way you are allowing this to open in your world. Although you know this also kind of affirms my legacy, from hearing you speak in the way that you do.

The first book is 'Black Issues in the Therapeutic Process' (2009). That book is based on the research, and the voices of those people involved in the research. The second book is called, 'The Challenge of Racism in Therapeutic Practice' (2016). This is more about actioning use of the concepts, that culminate in book three, 'A black Empathic Approach'-From Rage to Compassion.

I have described the steps that therapists can take to become robust in a black Empathic Approach. I have also shown that to achieve this model and make it their own needs reflection on personal development process and introspection about personal relationships with anti-black racism. Each chapter takes the reader through a process linked to this discourse, using transparency and my own life to demonstrate achievement of this model. It's over to you now.

Creating this legacy book has been like a rite of passage. I experienced blocks, silence and hopelessness about my ability and knowledge to present. On the other hand, I have experienced support and encouragement to see it through to completion. Here I am writing into the final pages and experiencing a sense of completeness. I have grown through the experience and learned a lot about myself and my ability to transform rage into compassion. I have been patient with myself when words failed me, and I learned that time can heal and bring about new feelings, loving thoughts and compassion.

October 2024

I spent the weekend with a large group of white people, members of the Reiki association. It was the annual gathering. I had anticipated that my internalised racism and hypervigilance would be triggered. Instead, I noticed where people approached me with a wish to engage, support and share parts of our lives. I held on to the direction we were given, 'to let Reiki lead'. There were times when I wanted to shrink away from some of the goings on and closeness. I connected briefly with a woman, who agreed that it was nice to see another person of colour, but we did not speak again after that. I noticed several women from various parts of Asia, Scotland, Ireland and parts of Europe. I enjoyed singing together, the hands-on energy sharing. I joined a music and movement workshop, in a small group led by Mel. I was moved to tears. I think it was because we were asked to work in pairs and in small groups, and mirror each other, touching hands and showing appreciation. For once I was not facilitating. I felt my vulnerability, having recently succumbed to some knee pain. I also felt appreciated and more connected to the other people in the workshop. I felt the compassion and acknowledgement of eleven others in the workshop, who were all white. When I returned home. I realised that I may have shed a piece of my hypervigilance, and I am sure this will contribute to living my compassion.

To all who read this book I wish you kindness, compassion and the self-care needed to transfer with grace, what you have learned from my journey and the sharing's and experiences of those who journeyed with me.

In remembrance of those gone before, such as Mary Seacole (1805–1881) dedicated Jamaican Nurse, during the Crimean war. Ida B. Wells (1862–1831) who was forced to the back of the Suffragette march and Marie Battle-singer (1910–1985) first black child Psychologist in the UK. Claudia Jones (1915–1964) Trinidadian journalist & Activist.

Bibliography

Akbar, N. (1996). *Breaking the Chains of Psychological Slavery*. US, Mind Productions and Associates.

Aleyne, A. (2022). *The Burden of Heritage*. UK, Karnak.

Alleyne, A., Tuckwell, G., Shears, J., & Wheeler, S. (2008). CD recording. UK, University of Leicester.

Andrews, K. (2023). *The Psychosis of Whiteness: Surviving the Insanity of a Racist World*. UK, Penguin Audio.

Andrews, M. (2013). *Doing Nothing Is Not an Option*. UK, Krik Krak.

Bailly, L. (2009). Lacan: A Beginner's Guide. UK, One World Publications.

Behrendt, L., Larkin, S., Griew, R., & Kelly, P. (2012). *Review of Higher Education Access and Outcomes for Aboriginal and Torres Strait Islander People: Final Report*. Canberra: Department of Industry, Innovation, Science, Research and Tertiary Education.

Clark, A. J. (2022). *Empathy and Mental Health: An Integral Model for Developing Therapeutic Skills in Counseling and Psychotherapy*. UK, Routledge.

Cooper, B. (2019). *Eloquent Rage. A Black Feminist Discovers Her Superpower*. Picador, New York, St Martin's Press.

Death of Orville Blackwood. (1991). Report of the committee of inquiry into the death in Broadmoor Hospital of Orville Blackwood, and a review of the deaths of two other Afro-Caribbean patients: "big, black and dangerous?". https://en.wikipedia.org/wiki/Death_of_Orville_Blackwood

Eddoe Lodge, R. (2018). *Why I'm No Longer Talking to White People About Race*. UK, Bloomsbury Publishing.

Franz, F. (1961). *Black Skin White Masks*. UK, Pluto Press.

Gemmel, O. (2020). *Why I'm Longer Talking to Black People about Race & George Floyd*. UK, Kindle.

Gilbert, P. (2013). *The Compassionate Mind*. UK, Robinson.

Hassan, K. M. (1999). *The Willie Lynch Letter & the Making of a Slave*. US, Lushena Books.

Hooks, B. (1996). *Killing Rage: Ending Racism*. UK, Penguin.

Keval, N. (2023) The Racist Gaze: Bearing Witness. In *Therapy in Colour*. UK, Jessica Kingsley Publishers.

Lago, C. & Thompson J. (1991). *Race, Culture and Counselling*. UK, Open University Press.

Lawrence, L. (2020). *The Louder I Will Sing*. UK, Sphere.

Lee, D. (2012). *The Compassionate Mind approach to Recovering from Trauma*. London, Little, Brown Book Group.

Lorde, A. (2007). Sister Outsider, Crossing Press. Penguin, Canada, in 'The uses of anger'. *Women's Studies Quarterly*, Vol. 25(1/2), pp. 278–285.

Mayfield, C. (1971). *Hard Times: Baby Huey*. Chicago, RCA studios

Mckenzie-Mavinga, I. (1988). *Charting The Journey*. Kay, J., Lewis, G., Landor, L., & Parmar, P. (Eds). UK, Sheba Press.

Mckenzie-Mavinga, I. (2003) Poem: *Christmas in Ghana*. Unpublished.

Mckenzie-Mavinga, I. (2009). *Black Issues in the therapeutic Process*. UK, Palgrave MacMillan.

Mckenzie-Mavinga, I. (2016). *The Challenge of Racism in therapeutic Practice*. UK, Palgrave MacMillan.

Mckenzie-Mavinga, I. (2020) *Dear Father*. (Dedication to Ernest Mckenzie-Mavinga son of freed slaves 1898–1948).

Mckenzie-Mavinga I. (2022). Poem: *Rain Forest Bathing*. Main Ridge Tobago. Unpublished.

Mckenzie-Mavinga, I., & Grant, A. (2023). *Therapy in Colour*. Carberry, K., Ellis, E., Black, K., & Mckenzie-Mavinga, I. (Eds). UK, Jessica Kingsley Publishers.

Mckenzie-Mavinga, I., & Perkins, T. (1991). *In Search of Mr Mckenzie*. UK, Women's Press.

Morrison, T. (1987). *Beloved*. US, Alfred A. Knopf Inc.

NourbeSe Philip, M. (2008). *Zong*. US, Wesleyan University Press & Canada, Mercury Press.

NourbeSe Philip, M. (2017). *Talk*. John Hope Franklin Humanities Institute, Duke University. www.google.com/

Patel, G. (2023). The Impact of Racism and Culture on Identity-a Psychoanalytic Intercultural Approach. In *Therapy in Colour* (pp. 244–255). Carberry, K., Ellis, E., Black, K., & Mckenzie-Mavinga, I. (Eds). UK, Jessica Kingsley Publishers.

Peele. J. (2017) Film *Get Out*. Universal Pictures. USA.

Pinkola Estés, C. (1996). *Women Who Run with the Wolves: Myths and Stories of the Wild Woman Archetype*. US, Ballantine Books.

Raleigh,V., & Holmes, J. (17 May 2023). The Health of People from Ethnic Minority Groups in England. UK, Health Inequalities, Public health, Equality and Diversity.

Rogers, C. (1959). A Theory of Therapy, Personality, and Interpersonal Relationships, as Developed in the Client Centred Framework. In *Psychology: A Study of Science, Vol 3: Formulations of the Person and the Social Context* (pp. 184–256). Koch, S. (Ed). NY, Mcgraw-Hill.

Ryde, J. (2009). Marianne Fry lectures. White Identity in Psychotherapy: Can dialogic, intersubjective psychotherapy help white people work more effectively in a racialized context? UK.

Samuel, N. K. S. (2023). A Thesis of Clinical Research and Practice: Part A: Disclosing Racial Trauma in Psychological Therapy: Exploring the Experiences of Racially Minoritised People in the UK; Part B: Cultivating Cultural Humility in Clinical Psychology Training: Bridging the 'Competency'/'Humility' Gap; Part C: Summary of Clinical Practice and Assessments [University of Surrey]. https://doi.org/10.15126/thesis.900841

Satre, J. P. (1943). *Being and Nothingness (2020)*. UK, Routledge, Marianne Fry Lectures.

Schultz, P. (2003). *1,000 Places to See Before You Die*. NY, Workman Publishing.

Tutu, D., & Tutu, R. M. (2015) *The Book of Forgiving: The Fourfold Path for Healing Ourselves and Our World 2015*. US, Harper Collins. www.betterup.com/blog/what-is-imposter-syndrome-and-how-to-avoid-i

Index

For Product Safety Concerns and Information please contact our EU
representative GPSR@taylorandfrancis.com
Taylor & Francis Verlag GmbH, Kaufingerstraße 24, 80331 München, Germany